Ethics of Newborn Intensive Care

INSTITUTE OF GOVERNMENTAL STUDIES
Eugene C. Lee, *Director*

The Institute of Governmental Studies was established in 1919 as the Bureau of Public Administration, and given its present name in 1962. One of the oldest organized research units in the University of California, the Institute conducts extensive and varied research and service programs in such fields as public policy, politics, urban-metropolitan problems, and public administration. The Institute focusses on problems and issues confronting the government and citizens of the San Francisco Bay Area, of California, and of the nation.

The professional staff comprises faculty members holding joint Institute and departmental appointments, research specialists, librarians and graduate students. In addition the Institute encourages policy oriented research and writing efforts by a variety of faculty members and researchers not formally affiliated with the staff. The Institute is also host to visiting scholars from other parts of the United States and many foreign nations.

A prime resource in its endeavors is the Institute Library, with more than 350,000 documents, pamphlets and periodicals relating primarily to government and public affairs. The Library serves faculty and staff members, students, public officials and interested citizens.

The Institute publishes books, monographs, bibliographies, periodicals, working papers and reprints for a national audience, as well as the Institute bulletin, the *Public Affairs Report,* which is issued six times a year. In addition, Institute-sponsored lectures, conferences, workshops and seminars bring together faculty members, public officials and citizens. These publications and programs are intended to stimulate thought, research, and action by scholars, citizens and public officials on significant governmental policies and social issues.

HEALTH POLICY PROGRAM
Philip R. Lee, M.D., *Director*

The Health Policy Program was formed in 1972 with support provided by the Robert Wood Johnson Foundation and the University of California, San Francisco. The program's purpose is to serve as an interdisciplinary resource group for health policy decision makers. A specific objective is to consider the problems of health care from the multiple points of view that exist in a complex society. Another is to change the climate in which public decisions are made—from what has often been an adversary process to that of an educational process.

Established as an integral part of the School of Medicine, the program's university base allows for training of students and exchange of information and ideas among a broad range of health professionals. It is the only major interdisciplinary health policy program based within a school of medicine on a health sciences campus.

Principal areas of study include primary care and health manpower policies, paying for medical care and controlling costs, quality of care assessment, the balance between medical care and other health measures, and bioethics and societal values. Ethical questions are given particular emphasis in the consideration of all policy issues.

Ethics of Newborn Intensive Care

Edited by
ALBERT R. JONSEN
and
MICHAEL J. GARLAND

A Joint Publication of
HEALTH POLICY PROGRAM, School of Medicine
University of California, San Francisco
and
INSTITUTE OF GOVERNMENTAL STUDIES
University of California, Berkeley
1976

The editors thank the Robert Wood Johnson Foundation and the Henry J. Kaiser Family Foundation for funds that contributed significantly to the preparation and publication of this book.

LIBRARY OF CONGRESS CATALOGING IN PUBLICATION DATA
Main entry under title:

Ethics of newborn intensive care.

Based on materials presented at conference organized by the Health Policy Program and the Dept. of Pediatrics, School of Medicine, University of California San Francisco, in May 1974.
    Includes bibliographical references.
    1. Neonatal intensive care--Moral and religious aspects--Congresses.   I. Jonsen, Albert R.   II. Garland, Michael J.   III. University of California San Francisco. School of Medicine. Health Policy Program.   IV. University of California San Francisco. Dept. of Pediatrics.
[DNLM: 1. Ethics, Medical--Congresses.   2. Infant, Newborn, Diseases--Therapy--Congresses.   3. Intensive care units--Congresses.   4. Critical care--In infancy and childhood--Congresses.   W50 E845 1974]
RJ253.5.E83   174'.2   76-47016
ISBN 0-87772-216-1

$4.00

This publication is distributed by the Institute of Governmental Studies

CONTENTS

PART II

The Social Context

PART III

Questions of Policy

THE DEFECTIVE NEWBORN: AN ANALYTIC FRAMEWORK
FOR A POLICY DIALOG

F. Raymond Marks with Lisa Salkovitz

FOREWORD

How, when and for what purposes should we employ
the science and technology that burgeon in our times?
For example, when should medical technology be used to
its fullest in trying to keep a threatened infant alive,
and when does the baby's probable future hold such grim
prospects that it becomes more ethical and humane to
withhold heroic measures?

Finding appropriate answers to such difficult questions in our fast-changing world is one of mankind's
most troubling endeavors. From the global scale of world
affairs to the narrow confines of a hospital, we see a
compelling need for prompt, realistic and pragmatic
decisions on the use of technology.

We need to make humane judgments that recognize the
consequences for all whose lives are likely to be affected. Time runs inexorably, crises recur, and irre-
versible decisions must inevitably be made under pressure because inaction is itself a fateful choice. The
burdens are heavy for those in roles of responsibility
and trust.

"Neonatal intensive care." The words standing
alone have an abstract, aseptic sound. The layman may
find that, like many medical terms, they mask the painful realities of daily life in a hospital. As Albert
R. Jonsen notes in the opening essay of this symposium,
neonatal intensive care--i.e., providing specialized
medical treatment for newborn babies who may be desper-
ately ill--is itself a newcomer to medicine and nursing.

In part because such care is new and rapidly changing, no accepted body of principles has been developed
to guide its use. Recognizing this, the Health Policy
Program and the Department of Pediatrics, both of the
School of Medicine, University of California, San Francisco, organized a conference in May 1974 to explore the
ethical issues and some of the policy implications of
neonatal intensive care.

The initial versions of most of the material appearing in this symposium were presented and discussed
at the conference. The material was subsequently reviewed and revised in the light of comments by knowledge-
able critics and editors. We believe that it makes
a significant contribution to the discussion and understanding of important ethical and policy issues of neonatal health care.

Accordingly, the Institute of Governmental Studies
is pleased to join the Health Policy Program in issuing
the results of the symposium effort. Moreover this publication furthers one of the Institute's principal ob-
jectives: encouraging better public awareness and understanding of policy implications that may be drawn from
research and related activities conducted or sponsored
by University faculty and researchers.

The symposium's contributors approached the common
topic with their several different backgrounds in pediatrics, nursing, economics, social welfare, psychology,
law, philosophy and theology. Each brought his or her
own discipline, knowledge, and experience, as well as
the philosophical, ethical and religious predispositions
that influence one's judgments in such matters. The
sensitive reader can weigh, compare and evaluate the
various views of the participants, which are often expressed tentatively and phrased to provoke further thought,
rather than stated as settled conclusions.

In short, the symposium did not attempt a definitive
treatment of its complex subject. The authors sought to

raise and explore the principle ethical and policy issues facing parents, families, physicians, nurses and other responsible persons who must participate in life-or-death decisions.

We wish to thank the symposium's contributors and editors for their careful attention to the successive drafts. We especially appreciate the diligent, unflagging care that Michael Garland gave to his "editorial brokering" role, working with our Institute staff, with his co-editor Albert Jonsen, and with the other contributors. Garland's persistent editorial effort and tactful negotiating skill were immensely helpful in bringing all the pieces together in this published product. Institute Editor Harriet Nathan gave the project her usual thoughtful attention, reading drafts, raising questions and supervising the final editing. Thanks are also due Lynette Ford, who typed the photo-ready pages, and Louise Gray who did the major share of verifying notes and references.

Stanley Scott
Assistant Director
Institute of Governmental
  Studies

Introduction:
Ethics and Neonatal Intensive Care

> The amazing progress of medicine is
> reducing more and more the dependence
> on nature and is enlarging the realm
> of human possibilities to change and
> correct the human condition....This
> is the reason why today we ask for
> ethics exactly at the point where
> nature or destiny previously reigned.
> The power of nature or destiny was
> blind. The power of man must be see-
> ing if it is to be human and respon-
> sible.
>
> > Jurgen Moltmann, "Ethics
> > of Biomedical Research,"
> > *Recent Progress in Bio-*
> > *logy and Medicine* (Paris:
> > UNESCO, September 1972.)

Neonatal Intensive Care is a recently evolved spe-
cialty in medicine and nursing. Work over the past ten
to fifteen years has yielded a considerable body of data
to guide scientific and technical advances in the medical
treatment of seriously ill newborn infants. A neonatal

Associate Professor of Bioethics, School of Medicine,
University of California, San Francisco.

1

intensive care unit brings together sophisticated equipment and specially trained personnel to provide the optimal environment for assisting the endangered infant through a critical stage in the transition to extra-uterine life.

Many conditions in the newborn require intensive care. A partial list of high-risk neonates includes:

those born of diabetic or drug-addicted mothers;

infants whose mothers suffered severe blood poisoning associated with pregnancy;

those born of Rh-negative mothers with rising quantities of Rh antibodies in their blood;

infants born by Caesarean section because of a variety of complications;

infants born after a prolonged labor, especially if the fetus has been in distress;

certain low birth-weight infants, whether born preterm or at term;

postterm infants (more than 42 weeks gestation);

infants distressed at delivery (e.g., respiratory distress);

multiple birth infants with potential problems;

infants with generalized infections (sepsis) or exhibiting post delivery distress (e.g., cardiac, respiratory, gastro-intestinal);

jaundiced infants;

and those with congenital defects requiring immediate treatment, such as heart malformation or gastro-intestinal blockage.

These problems afflict many newborn infants, killing 12 of every 1,000 liveborn babies and producing permanent handicaps in at least as many more.

The best estimates currently available suggest that at least 60 of every 1,000 liveborn infants will need some form of neonatal intensive care if we are to minimize death and disability. In the State of California, 9,000 to 10,000 babies required this sort of care in 1974. There are now about 20 major intensive care nurseries in California attempting to deal with these patients and each is repeatedly confronted with difficult ethical and moral decisions about who should receive intensive care and who should not.

ETHICAL QUESTIONS, PRINCIPLES, AND FACTS

This book deals with ethical aspects of neonatal intensive care. Most of the papers in the volume were prepared for a conference held in Sonoma, California in May 1974.[1] Here, as at the conference, we concentrate on such questions as, "Is it right or wrong to withdraw life-sustaining support in certain circumstances?" and "Who bears responsibility for such decisions?" We keep these questions of right, wrong and responsibility in mind as we pursue other related questions about legal status, cost effectiveness, realistic predictions of outcome, and familial involvement in life-sustaining activities.

Our basic questions are called "ethical" because they arise from and are answered by reference to ethical principles concerning rightness, fairness, equity and the like. The life-saving skills of intensive care teams have challenged our understanding of a venerable ethical principle in medicine: "One ought to save endangered life." Now the ethical question arises, "How shall we interpret that principle when it is possible to save the life of an infant so severely brain-damaged that he will never participate in 'human activities'?"

An ethical principle can be defined as a generalized normative judgment about behavior, based on values
arising from one's experience and beliefs and supported
by some degree of social approval. Persons offer such
principles as final justification for their choices and
decisions. Ethical principles exercise a ruling force
in the process of moral judgments, for we use such principles to weigh factual data. For example, the fact
of predictable mental deficit in a newborn child will
have different weight depending on whether one believes
that "One ought to save all endangered life;" or "One
ought not to inflict burdens on a family or society;"
or "One ought not to inflict the cruel life of a mental
retardate on an infant."

A statement by Gordon Avery, M.D., Chief of Neonatology at Children's Hospital, Washington, D.C., il-
lustrates the interrelation of ethical questions, principles and facts:

> Now we shoot for a meaningful life
> rather than how long we can maintain
> a heart beat. You always have to be
> helpful, not harmful. And there are
> times when to do everything you can
> is harmful rather than helpful.
> (Washington *Post*, March 11, 1974).

Presupposed in this statement is the ethical question, "Is it right to do everything possible to keep a
person alive?" Dr. Avery deals with this question by
appealing to the familiar medical-moral principle, "Be
helpful, not harmful." But the principle is only a
formality until given substance in relation to a specific view of the meaning of human life.

Supposing that meaningful life is defined as economically productive life, then saving those lives that
can be economically productive would "be helpful". It
would "be harmful" to save lives that cannot be economically productive, or not to save lives that could
be economically productive. Facts such as possible

mental deficiency and sensory handicaps, would be relevant to the ethical discussion because they are intimately related to capacity for economic productivity.
Other facts--such as capacity for delight and playful-
ness would be irrelevant to a discussion--but might be
of utmost importance if human values other than "productivity" were being considered.

Ethical principles are not always explicit in answers given to ethical questions. We believe it is important to deal explicitly with ethical principles so
they can be examined and criticized and evaluated in
the course of public discussion. While ethicists are
supposed to explain the meaning and set forth the justification of ethical principles, empirical scientists
must supply data relevant to the problem.

Thus the purpose of this volume is to facilitate
the efforts of health-care professionals and others
to understand, challenge and refine the ethical principles presumed relevant to neonatal intensive care questions. To this end, the book also includes empirical
data required to apply the principles to specific cases
and to project the consequences of acting on stated principles.

THE BASIC PRESUPPOSITION

This book takes as given the continued existence
and expansion of intensive care medicine for newborns.
We do not explore broad health policy issues that might
be debated, such as basic allocation of resources, and
priority of preventive medicine over crisis medicine.
These are not unimportant issues. They are left aside
for the moment only in the interest of dealing directly
with certain facts of life in contemporary American
health care delivery. Newborn intensive care units confront health care providers and consumers with the ethical paradox described by Wolf Zuelzer, M.D., who noted
that it is now necessary

> to consider whether and under what
> circumstances we might refrain from

> actively supporting [life] when
> the survival of an otherwise doomed
> child may be a greater misfortune
> than death. Having to make such
> decisions goes against the grain of
> a profession imbued with the notion
> of the absolute sanctity of human
> life, yet we cannot shirk the respon-
> sibility that comes to us from having
> taken the biological fate of man into
> our own hands.[2]

POLICY QUESTIONS

Should there be an explicit policy on the use of intensive care techniques?[3] Is an explicit policy contrary to good clinical practice, where each case should be dealt with on its own terms?

If there is to be a policy, should it be conceived in terms of a cost-benefit ratio? How much cost, in terms of energy, effort, time and money is justified by the outcomes?[4]

If outcomes are significant for the decision, how can one detect early signs[5] that would make it possible to determine when care is reasonable, with the likelihood of a good outcome? Are there, or should there be, definite criteria for initial resuscitation, for continued care, and for surgical repair of anomalies?

If there is some agreement on criteria for reasonable care, what is to be done when life-sustaining care is judged unreasonable? Should we let nature take its course? Should we intervene actively and directly to terminate life--active euthanasia?

NECESSARY DETERMINATIONS

In discussing these questions, the following determinations would seem to be essential elements of a pattern of ethical reasoning. Putting them together in certain ways would lead to certain conclusions, as exemplified below in the moral policy paper.[6]

1. Who are the parties in the case and what are their rights? This is stated broadly in order to include the baby, who is not a decision-maker but is affected by the decision, and others, such as the taxpayers, who are parties only remotely.

2. Who are the relevant actors and what are their responsibilities? This refers to all who may claim to have a part in the decisions. Their "responsibilities" are directly related to their part in the decisions.

3. What are the pertinent decisions each one must make or collaborate in? This refers to the diverse kinds of decisions: clinical, social,[7] economic, legal, which arise in the course of initiating, continuing, or possibly terminating care.

Note that none of the above three elements is equivalent to the frequently raised question, "Who will make the decision?" The really essential question is, "What are the principles on which anyone, whoever he is, should make a decision?"

4. What are the guiding ethical principles for this sort of situation? What is their precise meaning and their justification? Principles commonly accepted as relevant include: One ought to save and prolong life; one ought to effect maximum possible health; one ought to alleviate suffering; one ought not to do harm.

5. What are the clinical, social, economic and legal facts required to evaluate the status of care, both in general and in particular cases?

6. Finally, most important perhaps and most elusive, what are the underlying values that determine our acceptance and interpretation of principles? These include society's values and views of infants and children, of

human suffering, of mental deficiency or other handicaps, of the power and uses of technology, of the deployment of the community's resources, of the role of the healing professions, and of future population levels, among other things.

The following papers explore other elements in the ethical paradox confronting neonatal intensive care. The volume is offered in the belief that explicit discussion of the issues, although sometimes troubling, will be of assistance to health professionals engaged in neonatal intensive care, to parents of defective newborns, and to those responsible for administrative and policy decisions affecting neonatal intensive care units.

PART I

The Clinical Reality

Treatment decisions in the intensive care nursery are technically and socially complex. The three chapters in this part focus on the clinical world where the decisions are made.

First William Tooley and Roderic Phibbs, pediatricians specializing in neonatal intensive care, offer a brief review of the major developments in their field, particularly during the past fifteen years. In this period there have been significant advances in the scientific understanding of the transition to extrauterine life and in the technical ability to support critically ill infants. In the wake of the technical advances, questions have arisen concerning the wisdom of applying the technology in certain instances.

The second chapter is the edited transcript of a panel discussion involving several young health professionals. The panelists discuss three cases typical of those in an intensive care nursery. The discussion offers insight into the process of decisions to continue or withhold therapy as perceived by residents, interns and nurses.

In the third chapter Clement Smith, long a national leader in the field of pediatrics, reflects on the problems rising from neonatologists' increasing capacity to restore and support vital functions in endangered infants.

Although these problems can be viewed in wider contexts, inescapably it is in the immediate clinical setting that medical care professionals must deal with the convergence of their technological expertise, their personal values and their professional responsibilities to the infants and their families. The clinical context constitutes the first frame of reference for this study.

Neonatal Intensive Care:
The State of the Art

William H. Tooley[*]

and

Roderic H. Phibbs[†]

Facilities for intensive care of sick newborn infants have increased rapidly in the past 15 years. Growth in knowledge of patho-physiologic processes and consequent technical developments have made it possible to diagnose and treat infants who were beyond treatment only a relatively few years ago. Many of the techniques of neonatal intensive care have been borrowed from adult intensive care units and adapted to the size and special needs of the small newborn infant. Development has not always been smooth and, in fact, there have been many false starts and serious errors. However, progress has been steady, resulting in rapidly declining mortality and morbidity rates.

The first treatment center designed for the newborn infant appeared early in this century. It had separate rooms for mature and prematurely born infants, with

[*]Professor of Pediatrics, School of Medicine, University of California, San Francisco.

[†]Associate Professor of Pediatrics, School of Medicine, University of California, San Francisco.

11

special features to protect the small but essentially
normal newborn infant from a hostile environment. Since
most infant deaths at that time were caused by infection
or malnutrition, these units focused on providing adequate nutrition, maintaining body temperature, and pro-
tecting from infection.

In the 1930's it was noted that most deaths were
associated with frequent cessation of breathing (apnea).
Respiratory stimulants and oxygen were used in treatment.
In the early 1940's, improved incubator design allowed
the use of greatly increased environmental oxygen concentrations, but by 1954 high oxygen concentrations were
found to be related to blindness caused by retrolental
fibroplasia. In the mid-1950's oxygen use, and to some
extent intensive care, were curtailed. With this, the
mortality rate for infants with birthweight less than
2500 grams (5 1/2 lbs.) appeared to increase. For
example, in California, death from cardiopulmonary failure (hyaline membrane disease) reached 60 percent in
affected infants. Pulmonary collapse and failure of
the heart and lungs to function adequately were recognized
as the leading cause of death in the first month of life,
and there was a surge of research on cardiopulmonary
biophysics and physiology in the fetus and newborn infant. As new information became available, infants with
hyaline membrane disease were treated more vigorously.

By 1970, there were many new methods for treating
newborn infants. These included continuous monitoring
of fetal heart rate and uterine pressure to detect fetal
distress, and amniocentesis (analysis of the chemical
composition of amniotic fluid) for the diagnosis and
prenatal treatment of fetal disease, such as that resulting from Rh incompatability between mother and fetus
(erythroblastosis fetalis). Infant intensive care centers
used extensive monitoring of blood gases and chemistries,
as well as continuous monitoring of blood pressure, heart
rate and rhythm, breathing rate and pattern. Nursing
hours per day for each sick infant increased. Physicians
intervened aggressively to correct abnormal laboratory
values (e.g., low oxygen or low sugar concentrations in the

infant's blood) in an effort to prevent progressive disease. With the evolution of these new devices and techniques and the demonstration that they could cause a decrease in mortality, they were widely applied throughout the country and mortality from hyaline membrane disease dropped from 60 percent to 20 percent of affected infants. Simultaneously, mortality from other diseases of the newborn also declined.

It is generally believed that intensive care has been a major factor in the following dramatic changes in mortality rates. Between 1964 and 1974, the neonatal mortality rate (deaths under 28 days of age) in the United States declined from 17.9 deaths per 1,000 live births to 12.1 per 1,000 live births. Further, improved survival rates have been particularly notable for very small, prematurely born, "high risk" infants. During the past decade in New York City, the mortality in this group has declined by 40 percent. At the University of California Medical Center in San Francisco, a similar decrease in mortality has occurred, as shown in Figure 1.

Some newborn infants are likely to develop severe neurological deficits, and premature birth is the process most frequently associated with increasing the possibility of neurologic handicap. Most of the early reports on the development of small preterm infants were gloomy. Drillien[1] and Lubchenco[2] reported particularly disheartening results. Two-thirds of Lubchenco's subjects who weighed 1500 grams (3 1/2 lbs.) or less had serious problems. Hearing loss, decreased vision, mental deficiency, and cerebral palsy were common. Questions were raised about the wisdom of using intensive care technology to save the lives of infants who would survive as seriously handicapped persons.

Analysis from the collaborative project for cerebral palsy showed that neurologic abnormalities were more frequent in children who survived respiratory distress than in those who had no respiratory distress. [3] On the other hand, Stahlman[4] found the outcome for

14

INFANTS WITH BIRTH WEIGHT OF
750-1500 GRAMS (1.75-3.50 lbs.)
BORN AT U.C. MEDICAL CENTER 1965-74

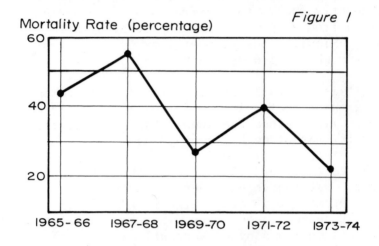

Mortality Rate (percentage)   *Figure 1*

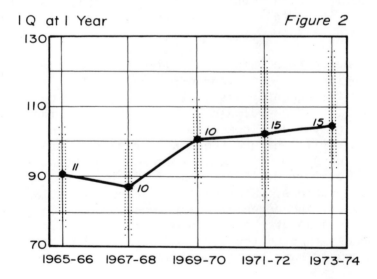

IQ at 1 Year   *Figure 2*

Note that mortality has decreased from approximately 50 percent to 25 percent over the decade while the average IQ of the survivors (as measured by the Cattell Test of Infant Intelligence) has risen from approximately 92 to 104. (The small dots show the range in IQ scores.)

preterm infants with respiratory distress primarily related to birthweight, independent of severity of disease.
This outcome suggested a positive effect from intensive
care. More recently, Lubchenco[5], as well as Stewart
and Reynolds[6] and Fitzhardinge and Ramsay[7], suggested
that intensive care has improved the quality of survivors.

These reports and our own experiences indicate that
when sick newborn infants, born with one or more conditions that threaten life or lead to an increased risk
of brain damage, receive intensive care they have a good
chance of surviving intact neurologically. We have been
encouraged by the dropping mortality rate but have been
aware of our obligation to determine whether the survivors are normal, since improved survival is not an advance unless accompanied by proportional decrease in
survivors with handicaps. Fortunately, our experience
indicates that the number of newborn intensive care
survivors handicapped by severe neurologic deficits is
also on the decline, as shown in Figure 2, for infants
of very low birth weight.

However, as medical science has developed techniques
increasing the ability to breathe for the non-breathing
infant and to restore the heart's action when the heart
is not beating, we find that occasionally an infant is
resuscitated who has already suffered irreparable damage.
Some infants with severe problems in the neonatal period
can be kept alive for long periods of time after it is
evident that there is no hope for long-term survival,
much less neurologically intact survival. This inevitably raises questions about the desirability of saving
certain lives, e.g., those who have ceased breathing for
prolonged periods whether before or during the course
of treatment. The problems of when not to intervene
and resuscitate an infant at birth, and when to stop providing life support for an infant whose brain has been
severely and irreparably damaged present continuing
ethical dilemmas for providers of intensive care.

Critical Decisions in the Intensive
Care Nursery: Three Cases*

ALEX STALCUP, MODERATOR: Decisions made in the
Intensive Care Nursery have significant effects on us
as developing professionals, on the emotional well-being
and intellectual functioning of established professionals
who work in and around the nursery, the families who
eventually care for the product of the nursery, and of
course on the infants themselves. On an everyday basis,
those of us who work in the nursery or have something
to do with it are forced to make decisions that may well
determine whether a child is going to live or die, and
the quality of that life should the child live. A developing body of data suggests that one who has been in
maximum intensive care now has a better prognosis than
he would have had five years ago for normal emotional
and intellectual functioning. Nonetheless, at the moment
of decision, the prognostic data are difficult to apply,
and we often feel that we are deciding in something of
a vacuum.

In order to provide an idea of the nursery milieu
and the type of thinking and interaction there, a group
from the house staff and nursing levels will share some

---

*This is a transcript of Pediatric Grand Rounds presented
at the University of California, San Francisco, October
17, 1974. See note 1 below for list of participants and
contributors.

of their experiences and show the way they think when they are confronted with an infant who requires a decision with ethical ramifications.[1]

Three brief case histories in ascending order of complexity will be presented to demonstrate some of the ethical problems we face. Panel members will comment on what they would do at a given point, how they would intervene, and what norms would guide their decisions.

CASE NUMBER ONE

MODERATOR: This little boy was born at 28 weeks gestation (about 3 months prematurely), weighing 1200 grams (2 lbs. 10 oz.), to a 26-year old mother. This was her second pregnancy. Her first, 5 years earlier, resulted in a normal child. The present pregnancy was complicated during the first 3 months when she developed severe ulcerative colitis, requiring surgery (ileostomy: diversion of the excretory tract through a hole in the abdomen). The pregnancy was further complicated 3 days prior to the premature delivery when the amniotic membranes ruptured spontaneously and premature labor and delivery seemed imminent. The amniotic fluid surrounding the baby became infected, and the mother was treated by antibiotics beginning about 6 hours before delivery.

The medical team made special preparations to provide optimal resuscitation for the infant at birth. These were explained to the mother by a senior staff member from the nursery. She was feverish, in considerable discomfort, and extremely agitated. She specified that she did not want a premature baby because she knew they all ended up mentally retarded and crippled with cerebral palsy. Her strong request was "Just get it out and let it die, and let me feel better." The doctor explained that chances for premature babies living and doing well were now much better than in times past, and that prior to delivery it was impossible to tell just how sick or severely premature the infant might be.

She was informed that the infant could be extremely premature with very little chance of surviving, and almost none of surviving intact if it was given no treatment. Or, the infant might be much more mature than expected, in very good condition, needing little or no special care, and could be normal. Alternatively, the child might be somewhere between the two extremes and require moderate intensive care--hopefully, with a good outcome.

The doctor assured her that he understood her concern and that he and the nursery team would try not to do anything unreasonable. The mother took only slight comfort from this explanation but to some degree seemed to accept the circumstances and became less agitated; nonetheless, she persisted in not wanting the team to resuscitate the baby.

The baby, born soon thereafter, weighed 1200 grams and appeared to be normally developed for 28 to 29 weeks gestation. There were no gross malformations but the infant was moderately asphyxiated, and was covered with infected, foul-smelling amniotic fluid. Do you think we ought to resuscitate this baby?

EILEEN ZIOMEK, INTERN: Yes, for a number of reasons. A baby of 1200 grams at 28 or 29 weeks has a much better chance than many of these babies born weighing 700, 800, or 900 grams. On a weight basis, this baby had a reasonable chance. The fact that the baby was born through foul-smelling, infected amniotic fluid is not a contraindication to resuscitating the child; our routine procedure would be to put the baby on antibiotics. I would not consider that unreasonable treatment.

MODERATOR: This mother specifically stated that she did not want the baby to be resuscitated. Do you feel that she should influence your decision?

INTERN: At this point no, mainly because I feel that the right of the child to live is an equal right. The mother is feverish and sick herself and not really capable of making that kind of decision.

MODERATOR: Let us assume that you are 26 years old and a nurse in the Intensive Care Nursery, and are about to deliver a prematurely born infant. You have a fever. Having one healthy baby, you decide you are not going to have an unhealthy baby and make it very clear that you do not want this baby resuscitated. Could you argue a little bit about your rights in this matter?

LESLIE CAREY, NURSE: I am the one who is going to have to take care of this baby and to raise it. We are going to have to foot the bills no matter how long this baby is in the hospital. I have one healthy child, and there is still a big possibility this baby may have some abnormality. Those concerns are very real. However, the fact that the baby is a good size is in the baby's favor. Or, assume that before birth we have no way of knowing what condition the baby is going to be in and there are a number of problems as far as funding is concerned. Or, I am a single mother and have another child and feel that I don't want a child who is going to be sick or take up a lot of time.

INTERN: Your decision to take care of the child, once the child is born, can be made later. If you do not want the child, you do not have to take him. But simply not wanting the child to live because you do not want to take him, would not be enough reason for us not to take care of the child.

MODERATOR: Michael, would you like to summarize this discussion and take sides on the issues?

MICHAEL SIEGEL, SENIOR RESIDENT: I think that Eileen is saying that the child has a good change of living and, at this point, we cannot say how the child will turn out; therefore, we should go all the way. Leslie, as the mother, is saying that she has some real concerns about how the child is going to turn out, and she doesn't want anything but a perfect child who is going to be like her other child. I would side with Eileen in this case. We should go all the way with the child at this point.

MODERATOR: We are also faced with the dilemma that if we do nothing to resuscitate the child, it may still live and suffer more severe handicaps because of our lack of action at that point. When the baby's death is not assured, should we not resuscitate?

SENIOR RESIDENT: One of the things I hear Eileen saying is that it is all right to disagree with the mother so long as you are willing to commit yourself to supporting her and the infant after the child leaves the nursery. That's at least one modifying factor on some of the kinds of decisions we make, because we assume that when we make decisions in the nursery this is an act of commitment that extends not just for the time being, i.e., the 2 months that the child will be in the nursery, but for the time thereafter.

CASE NUMBER TWO

MODERATOR: Our second case is a girl born by Caesarean section after a 34-week gestation to a 30-year-old mother. She had an abortion previously, and also have given birth by Caesarean section to a live infant with severe Rh disease (anemia caused by antibodies from the mother which destroy red blood cells in the baby) who died 2 hours after birth. The amniotic fluid was sampled frequently during this daby's gestation because of the risk of Rh disease. At 32 weeks gestation there was a marked increase in signs of severe Rh disease, indicating that the child would not survive for long in utero unless treated. At 34 weeks gestation, the child was given an intrauterine transfusion. Three days later the baby's mother went into labor and an emergency Caesarean section was performed.

At birth, the baby weighed 1700 grams (3 lbs. 12 oz.) and had an Apgar score[2] of 1. She made no respiratory efforts, she was blue, limp, had no reflexes, and a very slow heart rate. She was grossly edematous (swollen with excess fluid); the liver and spleen were very large. Vigorous resuscitation was required. Her parents clearly

wanted this baby very much, since they had taken a great
deal of trouble during the gestation in the hope of bringing her to term successfully.

Resuscitation procedures were initiated; a tube was
inserted through her mouth to her wind pipe and she was
ventilated with positive pressure; and catheters were
introduced into both the umbilical artery and vein. At
5 minutes of age, while she was being ventilated with
oxygen, her Apgar score was still essentially 1. Her
arterial blood had an extremely low oxygen concentration
(20 mm Hg) and a high carbon dioxide concentration; her
blood was very acidotic, with a pH less than 6.8 (Such
blood conditions carry the threat of damage to the brain
if not corrected rapidly). At 6-1/2 minutes of age her
heart rate was still quite slow, under 100, and a large
dose of bicarbonate was infused; at 11 minutes of age
her pH was still 6.9.

Should we stop resuscitation on this child yet? She
is now 11 minutes old, with a pH of 6.9, not breathing
on her own and not well oxygenated.

SENIOR RESIDENT: No, because there are infants who
do come through periods of severe asphyxiation and do
well. Also, you know the parents are eager for this
child; that's another consideration. We do not have
enough information to say that this child is damaged, so
we should continue resuscitating her, at this point.
One of the big considerations would be the parents'
wishes, and they have expressed a desire to go all the
way with this child.

MODERATOR: At 14 minutes of age her heart rate was
120, she had an exchange transfusion, and her blood pH
was 7.03, which is still very acidotic. The oxygen content of her blood was improving, but she was still floppy
and not breathing on her own. She was still edematous
and had no spontaneous activity. Marty, should we stop
yet? This family wanted to have a baby, but is it fair
for us to give them a retarded baby?

CHIEF RESIDENT: That's asking a question that we face often. What is our role? Can we play God? Can we stop? Can we just decide that it is time for this baby to die? It might be time to stop. The baby has suffered severe acidosis for 14 or 15 minutes and we know that along with the other complications of Rh disease there is an extremely high risk that the baby will be damaged. On the other hand, the parents' wishes do very much influence our considerations.

MODERATOR: The parents said they wanted a baby, but I did not hear them say they wanted *any* baby. Do you still think we ought to go on and resuscitate this baby?

CHIEF RESIDENT: At this point I have serious doubts.

MODERATOR: Let us assume that we did resuscitate and that very shortly thereafter the baby began to improve. At 22 minutes of age her pH was normal; at 1 hour of age she was placed on a mechanical ventilator, moved to the Intensive Care Nursery, and improved very rapidly. At 30 hours of age she was breathing spontaneously and although still floppy, she could breathe on her own. At this point the tube was removed from her lungs and she was taken off the ventilator, gradually weaned down to 40% oxygen with no difficulty. Her umbilical artery catheter was removed at 6 days of age, and it appeared as if we had triumphed over her jaundice.

She again developed jaundice and required another exchange transfusion, during which time her platelet (blood cells required for clotting) count dropped. She appeared ill for a brief period of time but then seemed to do all right. Everything seemed to be going well until the 8th day of life when she was noted to have difficulty feeding and her head size began to increase rapidly. At 2 weeks of age, needle punctures were made through the openings of the skull and the cerebral fluid was sampled. Deisel-oil-colored fluid, i.e., old blood, was removed from the subdural spaces. At 18 days of age,

a pneumoencephalogram showed greatly enlarged cerebral
ventricles and the cortex of the brain was about one-
tenth normal thickness.

Leslie, can you tell me what the nurses might think
at this point about what we ought to do with this child
who was acidotic, asphyxiated, with a pH less than 7.00
for 20 minutes, and now has hydrocephalus, and a tiny
cortex?

NURSE: The nurses probably think that this child
is not going to be a good "save". Loving this child is
not going to help take care of a retarded child.

MODERATOR: As a nurse working in the Intensive
Care Nursery, do you think it is ever right to stop
therapy on an infant this far into life?

NURSE: Yes, if this baby stopped breathing for
some unknown reason and required a mechanical ventilator,
that would be the time to stop on this child. She had
been severely acidotic, the cortex is much less than
normal, the baby is floppy. She'll have to have a shunt
to arrest the hydrocephalus. The shunt could become infected; it might have to be repeated, and even then the
procedures probably would not be effective. Or, she
could live to one year of age then develop even more
problems and die.

MODERATOR: Could you think of some examples from
your experience where the medical staff has felt that
we ought to go one way in saving the baby and the nursing
staff felt the opposite? Or, is there usually a fair
unanimity among the various staff members?

NURSE: Usually there is a difference of opinion
about timing. The nurses may feel that efforts should
be stopped sooner than the medical staff does. When
you sit next to the baby for 8 hours and it doesn't
move and you see there are no real signs of normal baby
activity, you begin to feel it is time to stop. However, at this point the medical staff has not yet de-
cided on withdrawing treatment.

MODERATOR: Can you remember any instances where this has happened? What effect does it have on your functioning as far as you can feel the tension in the nursery? Have you been caught in the middle where the nurses and some staff feel that we ought not be vigorous with this baby and the other half of the nursery medical staff feel we should be?

NURSE: Usually, you are on one side or the other. It is a very interesting phenomenon because it grows very slowly. But it can be at 2 a.m., when the interns or residents are sitting in the middle of the room writing their notes and the nurses start asking, "What is really being done with this child? Where are you going? What are the plans? Do you really think this child is going to be a good child?" You talk about it. Many times it stops there, because the child will then declare itself one way or the other. Other times, though, it begins to involve the Fellows, and then the attending physician. Very often the feelings are split right down the middle.

I can think of one example in particular. The nurses were very attached to the child and some of them really felt that the doctors were not going all out, and the child eventually arrested and died. There was a lot of feeling that not enough had been done by the doctors. The doctors felt they had gotten to the end of the rope, that we had nothing more to offer this child. This was an Rh baby, similar to the one you described, who went 4 months before he finally started having a series of arrests from which we were unable to pull him back. The nurses, though, had developed an extremely strong attachment to this child. But very often the nurses see a floppy baby who never opens his eyes or just opens his eyes and looks blank, and they want action sooner.

MODERATOR: I ask these questions because I want to make clear how very complex is the process of making the decisions in the nursery. It is my conviction that it is not the ideal situation. Decisions are made not

only on the basis of available data but often on a complex of the emotions of the nurses and family, the frus-
trations and fatigue of house officers, and personality
problems between physicians and nurses. It is a very
human process that has a lot to do with what eventually
happens in the ethical sphere.

CASE NUMBER THREE

MODERATOR: The third case, a very difficult one,
is even less clear. This boy weighed 1000 grams (2 lbs.
3 oz.), was the second of twins, and was born after a
30-week gestation to a 35-year old woman who had excess
amniotic fluid. The other twin was liveborn but died
during the first week of life. Onset of labor followed
spontaneous rupture of membranes, and delivery was by
Caesarean section. At 1 minute of age the baby had an
Apgar score of 1 and was resuscitated vigorously. A
tube was inserted into his airway, his lungs were in-
flated, and catheters were placed in his aorta. At 23
minutes of age he was given a blood transfusion.

He had a very rocky course in the first few hours
of life. By 90 minutes of age he was breathing spontaneously for the first time. He was eventually moved to
the Intensive Care Nursery from the delivery room, where
he continued to have a difficult course. At the end of
1-1/2 hours it was judged that he had been successfully
resuscitated (by blood gas criteria) although he had extensive bruising over his scalp and had poor muscle tone.
Throughout the therapy of this baby there were communication difficulties with the parents, who spoke very
little English. In general, they simply went along with
the decisions of the doctors regarding the intensity of
therapeutic efforts that needed to be expended upon this
child.

At 5-1/2 hours of age, the baby suddenly became blue,
stopped breathing, and required vigorous ventilation
through the tracheal tube before he began to breathe on
his own. During this episode his blood pressure fell

and he received sodium bicarbonate. At 8 hours of age
he was again breathing spontaneously, but it was noted
that his red cell concentration had fallen to nearly half
of what it had been, and the soft spot on the top of his
head was bulging. His spinal fluid was grossly bloody.
It was assumed that he had suffered a massive cerebral
hemorrhage and he was given a blood transfusion.

At 22 hours of age, the red blood cell concentration
had risen. At 42 hours of age, he began to twitch, his
color became blue, he had full-blown seizures, and his
blood pressure fell to almost half of normal. He was
again resuscitated. Somewhat later it was noted that
his blood cell concentration had fallen to nearly one-
third the normal level. It was again assumed that he
had a large cerebral hemorrhage, and he was again given
a blood transfusion. Mechanical ventilation was continued.

Marty, when do you think we should have stopped
with this baby?

CHIEF RESIDENT: There are many times when we suspect an intraventricular (cerebral) hemorrhage, but do
not have good proof that it has occurred and, at that
point, become very concerned that this baby is going to
be more severely damaged, maybe hydrocephalic. In this
case, it is fairly clear that he probably had two bleeds.
One of the things that concerns me about an intraventricular bleed is wondering how many babies with bleeds we
do not detect because they appear normal.

This is the second twin; the first twin died and
the assumption is that these parents very much wanted
this child. We do not know that, of course. We do not
know how many other children they might have, or whether
that should matter or not in our decision. This comes
up as one of the things we discuss when making decisions.
At this point I would still continue.

INTERN: I would have stopped, because, not only
with the intraventricular bleed but with the history from

the time of birth to that point, this child's prognosis for any sort of useful life is grim.

NURSE: There are many times when we suspect that but cannot prove it, so we have no idea how many of these children make it. I would stop.

MODERATOR: This baby developed severe respiratory distress. Each time they tried to take him off the respirator, his carbon dioxide rose to dangerous levels, and he had to be put back on the ventilator. By 10 days of age it became clear that he had a large open ductus arteriosus (a blood vessel required in prenatal life which normally closes off during the first day after birth.) He was in congestive heart failure and could not be removed from the ventilator unless he were operated on to close the ductus arteriosus. What do the nurses think at this point?

NURSE: That he should not be operated on.

MODERATOR: But the decision is made to operate. He is now 13 days of age and still convulsing; he is limp, he does not move much.

NURSE: His fontanelle (soft spot on top of his head) is still bulging (indicating hydrocephalus). We would all feel that this baby should not be continued.

MODERATOR: At 13 days of age, the ductus was closed and he tolerated the procedure well; feeding was resumed on the 14th day of age. He was removed from the ventilator at 15 days of age; however, because of a rise in the carbon dioxide level he was put back on the mechanical ventilator on the 16th day. By this time, x-rays of the lungs showed severe chronic lung disease. His eyes were examined at weekly intervals and retinal vascular disease was noted at 2 months. The retina detached at 3 months of age, and fibrous tissue replaced the retrolental area by 4 months of age. He eventually became totally blind.

At 3-1/2 months of age, he was still on a ventilator. An attempt was made to wean him from the respirator but within 24 hours he became dangerously asphyxiated and severely acidotic, with a pH of 6.80. He was lethargic, the soft spot on the top of his head was bulging; his head was rapidly enlarging; his abdomen was distended; and he was twitching, cold, and clammy.

INTERN: I would stop.

MODERATOR: It was felt that he had acute cerebral edema because of the high carbon dioxide and he was once more placed on the respirator. When he was again spontaneously breathing 60 percent oxygen against a pressure of 10 mm Hg and maintaining satisfactory arterial carbon dioxide concentration, another attempt was made to wean him from the respirator. Five days later, he began to have irregularities of the heart, his breathing was labored, his carbon dioxide concentration began rising and in several days it was quite high. A few days later he had signs of congestive heart failure, premature ventricular contractions became more common, and he had a respiratory and cardiac arrest.

Leslie, you're the nurse and we have devoted 5-1/2 months to this infant; we have put everything into him and, although he is blind, hydrocephalic, and on the respirator, are you going to call the intern to resuscitate him?

NURSE: S-1-o-w-1-y.

POSTSCRIPT

The final paper of this book proposes a policy for making ethical decisions in neonatal medicine. It emphasizes that critical treatment decisions must be based on both medical and ethical considerations and that the physician is only the medical, not the moral advisor and expert in these decisions. The preceding panel discussion raises questions about who should be the medical expert in decisions about terminating or continuing treatment.

Much of the dilemma in these decisions comes from the uncertainty of prognosis in many infants. Some of the cases presented in the discussion illustrate this point. It is reasonable, I contend, that the medical expert should be the person with the most experience in neonatal medicine who knows the case intimately; this must be the senior neonatologist in charge. He or she is the person who has the most experience with these kinds of decisions and, more important, the most experience with the long term follow-up of very high risk infants.

The house officers in training should participate in the discussion so they can learn from the process. But it seems no more reasonable to let them give the final medical opinion than it would be to let their surgical equivalents give the final opinion on whether a person should have open heart surgery or a cardiac transplant.

This view is based not on theoretical considerations but on practical experience. When patients are discussed who might be candidates for withdrawal of care, it is common for the house officer initially to favor discontinuance of care because of findings which he or she incorrectly interprets as indicating a hopeless prognosis-- whereas the more experienced physician can cite examples of a happy outcome despite equivalent or even more grave findings.

The discussion at the Grand Rounds demonstrates the authentic concern that house officers and nurses have regarding ethical decisions made on their patients. If they are not to give the final word, then they must never be left in a position where they feel that they have to make the decision because no one else will. They should never feel "the neonatologist thinks this case is hopeless but just cannot bring himself to discontinue care." In such a situation, the house officer or nurse may in effect make the decision to discontinue care by subconsciously reducing the intensity and quality of efforts. Such a decision lacks the processes of consideration we believe essential for an ethical choice.

One solution to this problem is an open discussion of the status of each patient who might be a candidate for discontinuation of life-support care. If care is to be discontinued, fairness requires that those most immediately responsible for delivering it be fully informed of the reasons for the decision and be allowed to express their opinion on the matter.

If care is not to be withdrawn, it is equally important that those giving actual bedside care fully understand the reasons for this decision. The latter situation is probably more important, and the neonatologist in charge must be acutely sensitive to any casual discussions, or even vague intimations, hinting that someone on the staff feels it is inappropriate to continue the care of a particular patient. The minute this occurs, it is time to initiate an open discussion of the case. In a busy unit, such conferences may be needed at least once a week.

Roderic H. Phibbs

Neonatal Medicine and Quality of Life: An Historical Perspective

Clement A. Smith[*]

Neonatology has always had its ethical problems. In 1937, when I began to work in nurseries for the newborn, births of occasional infants so malformed that their indefinite survival was then impossible raised the same questions that arise today: How long (and how) was the inevitable end to be deferred? While such confrontations, perhaps less frequent then because therapy was more limited, were less openly discussed than now, for those who had to shoulder the responsibilities of decision, I believe they were no less painful. They did seem however, to require a good deal less debate and discussion.

In those days, when no charge was made for the hospital care of newborn infants, the factor of expense did not enter into discussions. This, like other aspects of what is now known as neonatology, has changed. My assignment is to trace briefly the historical development of such changes, including some that have introduced a new issue facing the neonatologists and obstetricians of today.

---

[*] Professor of Pediatrics, Boston Hospital for Women, Emeritus, Harvard Medical School.

One might begin by noting that those earlier (and fewer) pediatricians working with the newborn 40 years ago were not formally recognized as neonatologists. That designation awaited coinage of the term "neonatology" by Dr. Alex Schaffer in 1960 during a period of rapidly expanding interest in what (concurrently) became known as the "neonate." Subsequently, this included the fetus, and some people who like that sort of thing refer to the neonate and fetus together as the "perinate." In those earlier days, and the tendency lingers still, pediatricians taking care of newborn patients were concerned essentially with attempts to keep them alive through a critical period of existence. Not until about 1960, as more and more newborn patients were thus prevented from dying, did we begin to think seriously about what people began to call "the quality of life" for those lives we were saving.

FOCUS ON NEONATAL MORTALITY

Several factors have always tended to focus pediatric attention on the prevention of neonatal mortality. One was, very simply, that there was so much such mortality. Also, in every birth, even the most normal birth of the most normal appearing 7 1/2 pound 40 weeks baby, there was always that dramatic moment--sometimes those agonizing moments--when we scarcely drew our own breaths while waiting to see if the baby would draw his.[*] That one act usually meant not only survival for a few minutes but for life, and--statistically probably--a life of normal length and reasonable quality. So when respiration was delayed or difficult, or the infant particularly tiny and immature, or structural or neurological abnormality was apparent, we troubled ourselves far less about the quality of the infant's future life

------

[*]Masculine pronouns are used throughout to avoid the cumbersome "his/hers" and "he/she" and the even worse inference that infants have no sex. Moreover, neonatal mortality is greater in males.

than about whether he could be given any future at all.
Moreover, if we could not produce immediately effective
respiration and circulation, our cautious assistance
was aimed essentially at keeping the infant from dying
until he could make the physiological readjustment necessary to continue as a living infant instead of a physio-
logically displaced fetus. This he could usually do
more effectively, and probably with less attendant risk,
than we could do for him.

If a two pound baby of 30 weeks gestation could not
survive when drained of mucus and placed in a warm iso-
lated environment of extra oxygen, no procedure then
known to us seemed very likely to increase his chances.
And if he died (as he often did) we presumed he was, in
simple terms, unable to live. Indeed, post mortem examination usually revealed a marked immaturity of the
lungs, frequently associated with intracranial bleeding.
Each was enough cause for death.

These very small and very premature infants, though
fortunately few in number, naturally had the highest
mortality of any group of infants selected by weight.
They still do, but more of them now live--and most of
those who die now live longer--than they used to do.

An interesting fact, and one not often realized
by the beginning medical student or intern, is that they
are more likely than not to start breathing at birth,
but their inability to sustain the process brings about
its cessation. Whereas this used to occur within the
first two days, the techniques (and the dedication of
those equipped to use them) in today's special care
nurseries now tend to extend the duration of survival,
sometimes indefinitely. A natural consequence of this
phenomenon is the increasing desperation with which the
baby's attendants fight for his mere survival as they
see his life prolonged.

QUESTIONS OF SURVIVAL AND QUALITY

Modern techniques can offer an increased chance for both life and "quality," but any life-or-death struggle interspersed with the usual periods of interrupted breathing (apnea) in the first week or weeks following premature birth can be much more damaging to the nervous system or brain than had it occurred later in gestational and extra-uterine life.

The recently collected data of two groups of neonatologists in Birmingham[1] and Montreal[2] about infants of less than 1,000 grams (2 lbs. 4 oz.) and those of less than 1,250 grams (2 lbs. 12 oz.) birth weight, offer hope that intensive care methods may in time offer not only survival but the increasing possibility of quality as well. Yet the risk of producing only the one without the other is likely to remain.

Workers in Lausanne, who recently presented their results in premature infants with the common--and commonly fatal--pulmonary disorder called hyaline membrane disease (HMD)[3] frankly reported that their "intensive care techniques increased the risk of infection and iatrogenic (medically or surgically induced) complications." Sixteen of 355 infants (mostly small prematures) surviving hyaline membrane disease in the Lausanne special care nursery were left with cerebral palsy or other severe neurologic damage. Another unhappy result of increasing intensive care techniques appears in the following quotation from their paper:

> The introduction of new therapeutic measures has not only increased the survival rate, but also has delayed the time of death in a large number of cases. During the years 1961-1965, only a few deaths of infants with HMD occurred after 27 hours; during 1966 to 1968, 15% of the infants deaths occurred only after 72 hours, 7% after the first post-natal week; some even

survived up to 3 weeks. The figures
for 1969 to 1972 were 25% (surviving)
at 72 hours, 20% at 7 days, and still
3% at six weeks. If death cannot be
prevented this delay involves a tre-
mendous prolongation of anxiety for
the parents and represents a tedious
burden for the nursing and medical
staff...finally ending nowhere. Fi-
nancially it can be estimated that
this delay in the time of death has
cost $45,000 for 1966-68, and $250,000
for 1969-72.

Thus the neonatologist may well ask himself if he
should enter upon and continue vigorous treatment of
every small premature infant with ominous respiratory
or other difficulty. In addition, modern surgical and
special care techniques raise similar ethical issues
involving more mature, and even full-term, infants.

CAUSES OF INFANT DEATHS

Duff and Campbell[4] have analyzed 299 consecutive
deaths in the Special Care Nursery of the Yale-New Haven
Hospital. Of these deaths, 256, or 86 percent, occurred
during the course of active treatment. The largest
single cause of death in these 256 infants was the respiratory problem of extreme prematurity. Perhaps "inability to live" describes the state of such infants,
and probably that of many others among the 256.

But in the other 14 percent of the total (43 infants)
death was "associated with discontinuance or withdrawal
of treatment." These infants were :

15 with multiple anomalies;

8 with trisomy (genetic anomalies usually incompatible with prolonged survival);

8 with cardiopulmonary problems (mostly associated
with prolonged treatment of HMD);

7 with meningomyeloceles (protrusion of the spinal
cord through vertebral defect);

3 with other central nervous system defects;

2 with bowel anomalies.

Survival of these babies could presumably have been further prolonged, but in the words of Drs. Duff and Campbell,
"like many others these children eventually acquired 'the
right to die'." For some of them the difference between
life and death may have been only the withholding of a
surgical operation.

SUMMARY

Modern knowledge, surgical skill, instrumentation
and the application of these in the modern special care
or intensive care nurseries, are increasingly successful
in preventing neonatal death. They are less capable--
and sometimes clearly incapable--of offering what most
people would call a life of acceptable quality in its
stead. The longer what were once unpreventable (and
usually early neonatal) deaths are deferred by modern
methods and the more another factor--that of expense--
enters the problem, the less acceptable is any course
except continuation of the treatment.

The writer offers only the final comment that any
universally applicable rule (except, perhaps, the Golden
one) for meeting these ethical issues is unlikely to be
attainable.

PART II

The Social Context

The second part focuses on the larger social contexts that influence or are themselves affected by
neonatal clinical decisions. Quality of future life
is an issue that cannot be avoided in the case of a
possibly brain damaged neonate. Psychologist Jane
Hunt addresses the question of how early one may accurately predict the impact of prenatal and neonatal
distress on later psychological development. Next
Marianna Cohen, a medical social worker, discusses
certain aspects of parental involvement in decisions
to prolong a sick infant's life. While it seems most
appropriate that parents be involved in such decisions,
they take place in highly charged situations in which
stages and process must be treated with sensitivity.

In the eventuality of a poor outcome--a living
but seriously impaired and handicapped child--the
family is faced with making provision for long-term
care and special education. In the third chapter,
Philip Lee, Professor of Community Medicine, and Diane
Dooley, pre-doctoral fellow in Health Policy, describe
the public programs available to support and assist
families thus burdened. On the level of public policy,
the existence, quality and accessibility of these
programs are essential aspects of the evaluation of
neonatal intensive care within the total health care
delivery system.

In the final chapter of this section, economist
Marcia Kramer addresses the question of the costs of

providing neonatal intensive care. Her analysis includes considerations of the cost of long-term care.

Through these chapters we are widening the circle
of considerations necessary for appraising the ethics
of neonatal intensive care. In the center of the
circle there is the medical professional applying the
fruits of science and technology to a sick infant.
But this would be an unreal and totally inadequate
picture without including the full range of social
influences upon and consequences of the technical,
clinical decisions.

Mental Development of the Survivors of Neonatal Intensive Care

Jane V. Hunt[*]

As the concept of intensive care for newborn infants has advanced over the past decade, important questions have arisen concerning the possibility of mental defects in patients receiving this care.

QUESTION I:

By using intensive care for children who would probably otherwise die, are we producing increasing numbers of mentally retarded or significantly handicapped individuals?

To evaluate the development of children who have received intensive neonatal care, a number of longitudinal studies have been instituted in centers in this country and abroad.[1] Reports to date indicate that centers that have provided intensive care for a number of years have experienced improved survival rates and, in recent years, reductions in the number of survivors with mental retardation and other severe neurological handicaps.[2] Neonatal care has dramatically improved

---

[*] Research Psychologist, Institute of Human Development, University of California, Berkeley.

the outcome for very small preterm infants, for those
who are difficult to resuscitate at birth, and for infants who develop respiratory and circulatory difficulties in the first hours or days of life.

For these groups we can say that the increased
rates of survival are not inevitably accompanied by an
increased incidence of handicapped children. In fact,
the reverse seems to be true. As methods in intensive
care have been changed and improved, the outlook for
normal development has also improved. The very small
preterm infants are illustrative of this trend. The
outlook for the survivors of this group was reported
as being generally poor in the early studies of the
effects of intensive care, but recent reports have
been more encouraging.[3] It is difficult to determine
the elements that contribute to these contrasting results because the studies represent a number of centers
with varying populations of infants. However, at the
University of California, San Francisco (UCSF), where
intensive neonatal care began in 1965 and has been uni-
form in its application since 1969, it has been possible to compare infants born in two time periods,
1965-68 and 1969-72.[4] Newborn care at this hospital
was improved in 1969 by the introduction of new techniques to combat respiratory failure, to control shock
and to improve nutritional status of the preterm infant. The results of the developmental test scores at
one year of age for these two time periods are shown
in Figure 1.

The number of infants with normal or superior development at one year of age has increased over time,
and the incidence of infants with poor development has
declined. Survival rate has continued to improve over
the years, but with an increasing rather than decreasing
incidence of normal outcome. Changes in intensive care
methods would seem to be the most important factor in
this observed difference.

The relation between IQ at one year of age and
childhood IQ is not perfect because some who do poorly

Figure 1

IQ DISTRIBUTION AT ONE YEAR OF AGE:
TWO GROUPS OF INFANTS BORN AT UCSF

(birthweights equal to or less than 1500 grams)

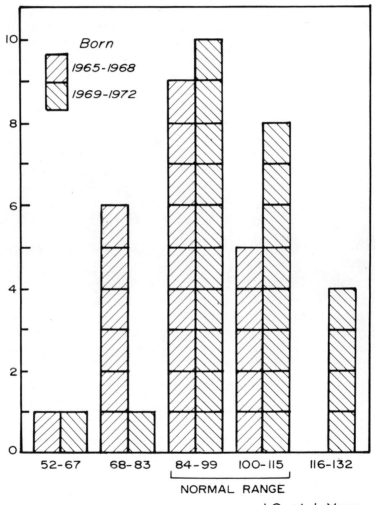

in infancy appear to recover and show normal development later. However, all the children who were retarded beyond the age of four years had below average infant developmental scores at one year of age. This leads us to predict that the more recently born infants will be relatively free of severe mental handicaps and our results to date support this prediction.

There are mental handicaps, not always evident in IQ scores, that impede some aspects of development in childhood and have an effect on school performance. These are the handicaps often referred to as "minimal cerebral dysfunction," such as language lags, learning disorders, distractibility, hyperactivity and emotional instability. These problems have been determined at ages 4 to 8 years for the preterm infants born in 1965-68. Figure 2 indicates these problems as being in the mild to moderate category. (The severe problems in Figure 2 are cases of blindness and, in one instance, cerebral palsy.) The high incidence of some developmental problems in the children with IQ's in the normal range is noteworthy. We do not yet know the incidence of these lesser handicaps in the more recently born children.

If, as it now appears, neonatal intensive care has resulted in a shift toward normality (i.e., fewer deaths and fewer retarded), then it is quite possible that this trend will also be reflected in the smaller numbers of children with minor mental handicaps. This can be determined as the children move into school age and as we work to develop better methods of assessing minor handicaps in infancy and the first years of life.

QUESTION II:

Are any of the methods of treatment now being used causing significant developmental problems?

The rate of survival for infants with some neonatal problems has improved dramatically because of specific innovations in care. One example is the group of infants

Figure 2

CURRENT IQ AND OTHER HANDICAPS:
28 INFANTS BORN AT UCSF 1965-68

(birthweights equal to or less than 1500 grams)

Number of Children

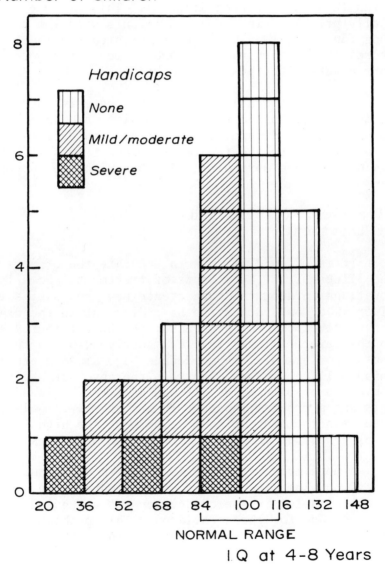

IQ at 4-8 Years

who had Rh blood incompatibility with their mothers and
were given transfusions before birth. Without this
treatment, these children either would have died before
birth or sustained severe mental retardation. Those
who had transfusions at UCSF have been followed closely
and are developing normally except for transient delays in speech development.[5] Another example is the
group who develop severe respiratory distress as newborns (hyaline membrane disease). This disease is especially prevalent in premature infants with immature
lung function. New methods of assisted ventilation have
increased the survival rate and improved the outcome
for infants with this problem.[6]

As each innovation in neonatal care is introduced
it must be evaluated for its immediate and long-term
consequence to determine whether any bad effects can
be attributed to the treatment procedure itself. Such
evaluations are more difficult than might be supposed.

Effects of Illness and of Treatment

It is often difficult to separate the effects of
the illness from the effects of treatment. Some innovations in neonatal care create new groups of survivors who would otherwise have died, as in the examples
above; developmental problems might be attributed either
to the severe illness that was survived, or to the treatment. For example, three decades ago small preterm
infants lived because of oxygen therapy, but had a high
incidence of blindness. It was at first believed that
this was a problem inherent in prematurity. Only years
later was the connection made between the high level
of oxygen given and the occurrence of blindness.

A more modern example is found in our group of infants who were given transfusions before birth. A
transient delay in speech development was noted at three
years of age for these children. This problem is more
likely related to their prenatal illness than to the

effects of the transfusions, considering the known results of the disease on the nervous system, but this assumption is hard to prove.

Treatment Practices Not Constant

It is difficult to relate a specific aspect of therapy to outcome when we find wide variations in the general level of care from center to center and from year to year at the same center. Changing practices in intensive care are ongoing and all are important to outcome.

Treatment Practices Individualized

Two infants treated on the same day at the same center may encounter different situations that cause different responses to a particular therapy. For example, for one infant we may have anticipated complications and have a medical team standing by at the moment of birth; for another, many minutes or hours may elapse before intensive care begins. Because of these variations in care we cannot readily speak of "the" effects of a type of treatment on mental development, but must examine specific practices and individual cases.

Treatment Practices Interdependent

Treatment for any specific condition may result in a series of decisions regarding the care of each infant. For example, the infant with birth asphyxia may have severe metabolic acidosis, which can cause damage to the brain. The treatment for this condition can be accompanied by a drop in blood pressure, which may decrease blood flow to the brain and cause additional brain damage unless blood volume is increased. A series of treatments is thus instituted, guided by previous therapy and the response of the infant.

Complications and
Brain Damage

Some of the complications that arise during an illness may be the most important determinants of brain damage. The complications that are the most devastating are intracranial bleeding, pulmonary airleaks, hydrocephalus, severe infection and congestive heart failure. These problems may occur with neonatal illness, and it is important to analyze treatment practices to see whether they are reducing or increasing the frequency of such complications.

Our research efforts to analyze the effects of specific treatment procedures must be guided by all of the considerations listed above. One way to do this is to look beyond the treatment to the infant's physiological state. The goal of intensive care is to normalize the infant's physiology, to stabilize him as quickly as possible and to keep vital variables within a normal range. We can examine the physiological state of the newborn and relate such measures as arterial blood oxygen and carbon dioxide tensions to the treatment used and then to the child's subsequent mental development.

Such analyses are underway at UCSF and a preliminary report has demonstrated the potential importance of this method.[7] We already know, for example, that the child's most abnormal value (e.g., his lowest arterial blood oxygen tension ever recorded) is not as important to mental development as is the time spent at the abnormal level. Consequently the rapidity with which physiological variables are returned to normal, and the successful maintenance of a normal state, are important considerations. In the future we plan to determine the relations between the time an infant is in an abnormal state and the occurrence of complications such as intracranial bleeding. Although the analyses of potentially damaging neonatal physiological states and their relations to later development are complex, they appear both feasible and necessary in order to judge the success of specific kinds of treatment.

QUESTION III:

How early in life can we determine whether or not an infant receiving intensive care has sustained significant and permanent damage to the central nervous system?

The time lag between the institution of new treatment methods and a full evaluation of their effects on mental development is of grave concern. In individual cases prognosis is usually not definite during the course of neonatal illness, often causing great anxiety. We can predict poor outcome with certainty during the neonatal period only when there has been devastating damage to the brain, with widespread destruction of nerve cells.

Some lesser degrees of damage that can be demonstrated by neurological examination of the newborn are not necessarily permanent nor predictive of developmental problems.[8] Some mild but permanent disorders are not readily demonstrated in early infancy, but may be seen in childhood as the learning and behavior disorder that we associate with minimal cerebral damage.[9]

Special Risks

Some categories of infants face special risks of developing mental abnormalities. For example, the very small preterm infant is at high risk for later problems. We know that these infants born at UCSF since 1965 have a better prognosis if they were born after 1969, did not develop hyaline membrane disease and were females. But, of course, there are always exceptions. We also know that high-risk infants fare better if they go home to a supporting environment. This is true for all infants and appears to be especially true for those who begin life with some potential problems.[10] The significance of the environment for subsequent development underscores the important effects of experience on brain development, even when there has been demonstrated damage.

Our longitudinal study of children who received neonatal intensive care allows us to examine developmental
data that were gathered beforehand for children whose
outcome is now known. As noted above, when we look back
at the early development of retarded and normal children
we find that by one year of age the retarded children
were already showing developmental delays. However,
some children who are now normal in every respect, and
a number of those who have mild problems in childhood,
were equally delayed in their development at one year.

It appears that if the infant is normal at one year
of age we can predict that he will not be frankly retarded from the effects of neonatal events, but if he shows
a developmental lag in infancy we cannot yet predict the
permanence or importance of the lag. More research is
needed to determine the significance of infant development for later functioning. We are currently following
the development of a number of infants by repeated tests
and measures during the first year of life, looking for
trends in development that can be related to neonatal
physiology, for sex differences, variations in family
environments and other factors in infancy that may improve our ability to predict later problems.

Assessment During Preschool Years

During the preschool years a number of developmental tasks are perfected to an extent that permits us
to diagnose moderate retardation with more confidence,
and to look for indications of some of the problems
that will cause difficulties at school age. Language
development and the acquisition of fine motor skills
are two examples of behaviors that can be assessed
during this age period. However, the problem of dis-
criminating transient from permanent disorders is still
evident. For example, infants who had received transfusions before birth have speech articulation problems
at three years of age. But by five years of age the

problem is much less evident, and mental development is normal, including language functioning. Whether other delayed effects will emerge at school age is not yet known, but there is no evidence to suggest that they will.

By four years of age the normal child's score on a test of intelligence is likely to be predictive of his future performance, particularly if his environment has been and continues to be relatively constant. The milder forms of mental retardation and other indications of brain damage may be determined with some confidence beginning at this age. This lag of at least four years from neonatal illness to the time when a reasonably accurate prognosis can be made of development of the mildly retarded and educationally handicapped represents the current state of knowledge. It reflects the complexities already considered in assessing brain damage from neonatal behavior and infant status. It also suggests the importance of the interaction between environmental events and development.

This leads us to a final question that is more likely to be posed by parents and educators than by those concerned primarily with the evaluation of intensive neonatal care:

QUESTION IV:

What are the remedial implications of a diagnosis of neurological disability?

If severe retardation is diagnosed in infancy, or moderate retardation is determined during the preschool years, or mild retardation and learning disorders are noted in early childhood, what are the remedial implications of these diagnoses? Must we assume a direct correspondence between diagnosis and prognosis? A strictly neurological model of cause and effect would assume that damage and disability are the same. A developmental model of behavior assumes the importance

of environmental influences in all cases of disability,
and research has supported this model by demonstrating
the plasticity and recuperative capacity of the developing brain.

In cases of minimal disorder, e.g., speech defects,
we may readily accept the proposition that a child can
be helped through speech therapy. We may also accept
the evidence now being put forward that children who
are potentially mentally retarded on the basis of familial or cultural deprivation can show improved rates
of mental development in response to massive environmental intervention.[11] But the child who is retarded
on the basis of known neurological damage is often considered a "hopeless case." Because diagnostic labels
often generate self-fulfilling prophecies we may find
considerable evidence to support this conviction.

However, by the time a retarded child reaches the
age of four or five years we are able to explore a range
of functioning and can usually demonstrate variability
in his abilities, just as we can for a normal child or
for one with minor disabilities. When we diagnose a
five year old child as bright or retarded, we are talking about an aggregate of functional abilities that we
group under the general rubric of intelligence, and
that we relate to his chronological age. His capacity
for further development is, of course, assumed. But
how he develops depends very much on the nature of his
ongoing environment and opportunities for optimal growth
in all the functions that we label "intelligence".

Potential and Present Performance

The child who is handicapped on the basis of neurological disability is of course different from the child
who suffers from cultural deprivation. But, for each,
there may be a wide discrepancy between present and
potential performance. This paper deals only with the
former category. The way the child responds to remediation is the best measure of that discrepancy, if the

remedial effort is directed specifically to the child's pattern of abilities.

For example, in one kind of reading disorder a child who is otherwise normal may not be able to discriminate among letter shapes. This inability is normal in the first few years of life, but in some kinds of mild neurological handicap the visual discrimination function is markedly impaired. There is a remedial technique for this in which the child learns to discriminate the letter shapes through kinesthetic cues, using raised letters. Once he can do this he often can proceed to the visual discriminations. We do not know how he makes this transition but we know that, without this special technique, his ability to make the necessary visual discriminations is profoundly delayed. Unless we understand the exact nature of his handicap and also know his better capacities we cannot expect to teach him to read. The developmental model of behavior assumes that his specific disability can be overcome by training that takes advantage of better abilities and, in many cases, subsequently leads to improvement of the specific disability. Such a model is quite different from a neurological one that diagnoses "dyslexia" and predicts permanent disability.

Under the developmental model we would consider the severely retarded child as one who has a nubmer of specific deficits and very few, if any, abilities intact. The remedial challenge presented by this child is greater but the philosophy is the same, as we work to find ways to advance development in a number of functional skills. The more severely the child is retarded, the earlier he is diagnosed, and the earlier skilled remedial help can be sought. Also, the more retarded the child, the more basic and life-enhancing are the skills that can be developed through remediation. Sometimes the results of consistent, sustained remedial programs are quite surprising. For example, in one research project a group of institutionalized children learned to read despite having Down's syndrome, a moderate form of retardation in which children are usually labeled "uneducable".

Environmental Variables

The range of environmental variables that are important for normal development in all children are also important for those with neurological problems. These include such disparate elements as nutritional status, opportunities for sensory and motor stimulation, social learning, language learning and the like. All children, whatever their age and handicap, are influenced by these environmental supports. However, the environment that would be considered adequate or optimal for a normal child may be less than adequate for the neurologically damaged child. For example, the usual environment may not provide sufficiently intense and directed stimulation. This would be true for a child whose primary deficit is an inability to learn from the normal or usual environmental events, and whose development reflects this lack of direct input. For another child, the usual environment may be overwhelming because, for him, there is an excessive and disorganized input. In both examples, parents and educators can work together to structure the total environment so that it supports and promotes development.

FUTURE RESEARCH

The task for future research is to continue to explore the relations between neonatal illness, practices of intensive neonatal care, newborn physiology and mental development. It may be possible to diagnose earlier in life some of the disorders that are now considered delayed effects. If so, the implications for treatment are good because we then may begin to intervene and normalize the course of development during the first years of life when mental growth is most rapid.

We know that some effects on development are transient, in that they seem to disappear during the course of development, while others are long-lasting. The differences may be attributed to the environment, and the

extent to which it is supportive in providing the means
to overcome the handicap, as well as the severity of
the damage to the nervous system. For children with
serious handicaps we may come to rely more on specific
programs of remediation as a diagnostic tool.

Ethical Issues in Neonatal Intensive Care: Familial Concerns

Marianna A. Cohen[*]

It is vital that parents of defective or critically
ill newborn infants be involved in the critical decisions affecting their children, because the parents are
the ones most likely to nurture the child in the long
run, and the first "set" of the parent-child relationship is crucially important to the development of their
later interaction. Whether we are discussing participation in the key decisions about how far to extend treatment, or only a truly informed consent to the physicians'
decisions, the parents' collaboration is imperative.

Parents show a wide range of individual reactions
to the birth of a baby needing intensive care. Many factors help determine these reactions, including social
class, life style, religion, culture, familial ties, in-
tra-psychic makeup, the special meaning of this particular baby, and others. But whatever their reactions, the
birth of a sick, premature or damaged infant is a severe
shock for almost all families. How and whether this
shock is resolved relates directly to the parents' opportunity to take part in the necessary decisions.

No one is able to participate effectively in rational decisions while under severe stress and tied up in

---
[*]
Medical Social Worker, Department of Pediatrics, University of California, San Francisco.

emotional knots from shock. For parents to play a meaningful part in informed decisionmaking, their initial
shock and denial must have subsided enough to let them
understand clearly the problems and choices confronting
them. It is in the best interests of hospital staff,
parents and infant for the evolution of their response
to be understood and facilitated as much as possible.

GRIEF REACTIONS

While the common range of parental reactions to
sick, premature or defective babies shows a wide variety
both of intensity and adaptation, the process by which
each parent moves from shock to adaptation goes through
a series of fairly well-defined stages. It is common to
us all, and has by now been quite clearly identified.[1]
The steps we go through in coping with a serious emotional shock have been documented in many different kinds
of grief reactions. These are denial, anger or depression, bargaining, acceptance and grief, and adaptation.
They usually occur in the order given with considerable
overlap, going back and forth, reviewing and reexperi-
encing. However, in the Intensive Care Nursery (ICN)
situation I have observed that, once through the initial
denial, the first run-through of the whole process takes
place within two or three days and the outline of the
final adaptation is often already set. This is the time
when intervention is most productive for arriving at the
soundest possible adaptation.

Denial of the fact of the baby's condition--that it
is alive, but sick or damaged--comes through in several
forms: in initial reactions with statements such as
"Take it back," "Don't let it live," "Everything will be
just fine," or very commonly a temporary, complete block-
ing out of the doctor's explanation of what is happening.
Occasionally there are continued distortions, but most
commonly the initial denial subsides into only occasional
feelings of "This isn't happening" or "It's not my baby,"
especially when the parents are encouraged and supported
in becoming familiar with the baby as it actually is--
tubes, respirator and all.

Anger and/or depression, which seem to be essentially the same feeling turned outward or inward, are the next stage and are often the hardest for the staff to deal with. Anger may take the form of a man's blaming his wife, the hospital, the obstetricians, the pediatricians. The object of the anger will consider it most unfair and probably respond with an exasperated defensiveness, unless the anger is understood as a "natural" part of the reaction that is being deflected onto doctors or nurses or the institution. Where staff avoid responding like a hit target, these feelings usually go on into efforts at bargaining, placating fate, and then acceptance of the sick baby, instead of the hoped for "healthy, bouncing boy." This acceptance then makes possible open grieving and mourning.

INITIAL SUPPORT

Overall, the most constructive handling of this situation seems to be a combination of supportive concern and involvement of the parents with the baby and with the reality of what is happening, as much as possible. When the hospital atmosphere permits open expressions of disbelief, guilt, depression, anger and grief, and provides good, clear, reasonably consistent information about the baby's condition, most families move fairly quickly to some adaptation towards the fact of this particular baby with its particular diagnosis. When the hospital situation is not conducive to such resolution, the process is much more complex and the number of unsatisfactory adaptations is greater.

Parents who seem blocked or hung up at any one of the steps in the process can usually be identified by continuing reactions that are either very much more intense, or much less intense than the situation seems to warrant, or by some continuing difficulty in taking in clear medical information. They appear either much too optimistic or pessimistic. Obviously this applies only when the information is clear and consistent. When parents appear blocked, they probably should have some

professional help with their grief reaction from anyone
on the staff equipped to give it: the social worker,
chaplain, psychiatrist, nurse, or pediatrician.

Any real involvement in either informed consent or
decisions about the baby's care implies the assumption
on the parents' part of some responsibility towards this
particular baby, and therefore is likely to occur only
when parents have moved past their initial shock and
denial to at least the beginning of acceptance. It may
be impossible to include them in decisions made at birth
when they are in shock, unless the possiblity of problems has been discussed in advance.

This process is complicated when babies are transferred into a central hospital from some distance away,
but it can often be accomplished successfully with a
combination of thoughtful planning and good, frequent
communication. There are of course some parents who,
under the best of circumstances, do not get much involved
with their babies; but even here real participation can
often be developed by communication, encouragement and
perhaps the inclusion of the family member who will in
the long run be the baby's caretaker.

INTERRELATIONSHIP OF DIAGNOSIS
AND GRIEF REACTION

No matter to what extent parents are involved directly in the ethical issues in an Intensive Care Nursery,
it is clearly important for the staff to be aware of
their reactions with the eventual implications for relating to the baby, and the nature of the community
options open to the parents. The wide range of parental
reactions, and the multiple factors that go into these
reactions were mentioned earlier. However, when I did
a retrospective survey of parental responses to all the
sick and/or premature babies born in our hospital in
1965, I found that by far the most common determinant
of initial parental response was the nature of the infant's problems. These responses had been recorded at

the time of the babies' illness, and were coded later for severity of reactions, appropriateness in terms of the illness itself and eventual resolution.

Variables of class, culture, and marital status seemed to have little effect on the nature of the re-actions, except that the relatively few parents with very unusual reactions also had serious emotional or interpersonal problems. The number of babies involved in this survey was too small for a definitive study, but the survey has proved to be a useful guideline for evaluating parental reactions.

(This section, which expands on the survey, is principally the result of several years of clinical experience. Originally done for my own learning, the survey was illustrative rather than definitive, and was not written up for publication.)

Prematurity

Gerald Caplan, in a study done at Massachusetts General Hospital,[2] identified the typical reaction of the mothers of premature babies as guilt. The guilt reaction is probably connected with feelings of failure through inability to carry the baby to term, is generally more severe when the baby is carried less than seven months, and seems often to be alleviated when the mother is encouraged to participate in the baby's care in one way or another. My survey included 24 mothers of pre-mature infants.

All of them expressed feelings of guilt and self-blame. However, there was great variability in the in-tensity of their reactions, in their ability to begin a relationship with the baby, and in the extent of their worry about the possibility of mental retardation. Twelve of them had serious trouble resolving their re-actions: five of the nine women with babies weighing under 1500 grams (3 lbs. 5 oz.) and nine of the fourteen primiparas (women having their first babies).

These figures suggest that the extent of the prematurity and the experience of the mother with previous pregnancies are significant factors in their reactions. To illustrate the variations there was, first, the young mother of an 1100 gram (2 lbs. 7 oz.) baby who sat on her bed crying, as she carefully and hopefully embroidered her baby's name on a bib. And, second, the mother who confided that she hoped the doctors would never let her take her 1200 gram (2 lbs. 10 oz.) baby home because she was afraid she would kill it.

By way of contrast it was striking in the survey that of the 17 mothers who had very small, but full-term babies (intrauterine growth retardation), only one expressed anything but loneliness and mild worry, and none of them expressed any guilt or self-blame at all.

Respiratory Distress

The parents of infants whose primary problem was respiratory distress showed little evidence of guilt, but considerable anxiety and grief. In only 3 of the 16 cases did the parents show anything other than this reaction. Typically, the anxiety would later resolve into grief at the baby's death or acceptance of his full recovery. Also, relatively few parents continued to act or feel overprotective toward the child by the time he had been fully recovered for several months.

There is one reaction that can be puzzling. Often when an infant is critically ill for weeks, with his survival uncertain, parents who have previously appeared to relate well to the baby, and to have handled their grief and worry appropriately, begin to sound either very pessimistic or very optimistic, no matter what information they are given. This suggests that prolonged, anxiety-provoking uncertainty is unbearable, and that the optimism or pessimism is a defense that will disappear when the situation is resolved, especially if the earlier reactions have been normal.

Rh Incompatibility

Families with an Rh problem contrast with the families of babies with respiratory distress. Survey families with an Rh problem, where the mother had received intrauterine transfusions during pregnancy, usually greeted the delivery of the live baby as an achievement. Especially in families with a history of stillbirths or infants lost, most mothers showed a high maternal drive, and the children were generally accepted, loved, and clearly much wanted. Of the 15 families studied, only two showed anything other than a combination of relief, pride and appropriate worry. The Rh children always have continued for years to be "special." They seem to be perceived as "a gift" and as sunny children to be loved for themselves. There has characteristically been a rather low degree of overt worry on the part of the parents about their speech delays or the possibility of mental retardation.

Genetic Defects

I have much less generalized information about the parents of infants born with genetic defects. Many of the infants in this category are transferred into our nursery, and they are seldom followed by us after their discharge. However, what observations I have suggest that this may be one area where the individual variations of parental reactions are among the greatest. Two examples may illustrate this. First, there was the very young father who, when presented with his baby who had a cleft lip, stated in shock, "Take it away; send it back. When you get a new car that's damaged, you return it to the factory, don't you?" And on the other hand, there were the loving parents of a baby born without a brain (anencephalic) who came daily to feed the baby as long as it lived, saying that they felt this brief experience of parenthood could be--and was--joyful and loving as well as full of grief and pain.

Retardation

The attitudes of parents toward infants who are expected to be retarded such as Down's syndrome babies,
also vary widely. There is the initial shock and grief,
well-documented in the literature,[3] but after the first
reaction, the responses are individualized. As examples,
there are the adaptations to four different Down's syndrome babies, born at our hospital. They were held in
the Intensive Care Nursery only briefly.

First, there was the intelligent, well-educated,
"back-to-the-land" hip couple. They reacted with open
grief, then loving acceptance. They visualized their
baby living a free, active, happy life in their rural
surroundings, and were not at all interested in long
range programs to develop the baby's potential to his
highest possible level.

Second, there was the Latin American couple. The
mother had hoped for a son, specifically to restore her
failing marriage. When an impaired girl was born, the
mother had a brief mental breakdown (postpartum psychotic
break), and the baby was placed in a foster home. The
marriage is now over; the mother has recovered well.
She is now actively developing both self-confidence and
economic skills, and says she is stronger and more content than before. She is affectionate towards the baby,
visits her, and brings her home to the older children
occasionally, but will probably never assume the child's
full care.

Third, there was the hard working, upward mobile,
lower middle class family who already had one mildly
impaired child. They initially responded with grief,
rage, and then despair. To quote the father, "Hitler
had the right idea, nobody wants misfits." The father
tried unsuccessfully to arrange private placement for
the baby out of the country. The mother is now caring
for the child at home, competently and sadly. The father
is quite distant and uninvolved.

Fourth, there was the young, stable couple who showed grief, then acceptance. They developed an immediate drive to train and educate their baby to the limits of his ability. They pushed for information, for books to read, for stimulating exercise programs, for every available community facility, and in general for whatever knowledge would help them develop their baby as much as possible.

LONG TERM IMPLICATIONS

Obviously, the parents of very ill or very premature babies usually worry about whether the baby, if he survives, will be slow and/or brain damaged. Families differ greatly in the emphasis they place on intellectual function; this emphasis affects their participation in the difficult decisions to be made in the ICN. Frequently the extent of the impairment may not be known for years, leaving the anxiety unresolved.

The degree and nature of the child's handicap is, of course, crucial to the long run adaptation. When the handicap is severe, I can think of no instance where the child has not proved to be a major and continuing disruptive force in the family's life. Where the handicap is moderate, and the child relates normally (some seriously brain-damaged children do not), some families accept the children as they are. Others in similar circumstances deny any awareness of the problem until the children reach school age, when the parents' anguish can be severe as they again confront the failure of their hopes. When the child is only a little slow or minimally brain-damaged, most families tend to remain unaware of problems until school age, and to deal with them then primarily in terms of family goals, or their aspirations for that particular child. Some families value warmth and emotional interaction more than academic ability; some accept whatever happens as their fate, while many grieve all over again as they recognize the child's limitations.

COMMUNITY RESPONSIBILITY

It is important to remember that those families whose child survives as a moderately or severely impaired individual will continue to need some community help in raising the child, no matter how well they have come to terms with his or her handicap. Ideally there should be a wide range of options to meet the needs of many different families and children: special schooling, respite care (brief, out-of-home relief care), out-of-home placement, counselling, and so forth. Most states mandate the provision of some special school facilities, but both the availability and the quality vary widely.

In California there is now a widespread network of regional centers to offer supportive assistance to such children and their families. At the same time, possibilities for placement out of the home, never abundant, have become more limited. Many states probably have considerably less to offer than California, and in all of them programs are subject to the yearly fluctuations of state budgets and state commitment.

In the absence of a deep, ongoing, overall sense of community responsibility and support to these children and their families, while making decisions we need to remember that the long term costs--financial, social, emotional--are likely to be heaviest for the families themselves. There is an old custom, in several cultures, that he who saves a life is responsible for that life. The decisions made in an intensive care nursery affect the child, the family, the state, the physicians, and other staff. But if the child is handicapped, who assumes responsibility for care? Usually the family does, sometimes the state does, but never the physicians and the hospital. That is why I think the hard decisions, while they should be medically sound, cannot be unilateral. Families must be involved to the best of their ability, and increasingly families are demanding this right.

Social Services for the Disabled Child

Philip R. Lee[*]

and

Diane Dooley[†]

Intensive care for newborns has prompted increased concern for the quality of life for those who have been saved. Most of the survivors of neonatal intensive care will suffer no handicapping aftereffects and their quality of life determinants will be those of a normal child. Yet for some, those who are born with serious congenital defects, or who develop physical or emotional handicaps as the result of prematurity, respiratory failure or other problems, an important determinant is society's response to their problems. The social, financial and medical resources that can be mobilized for long term care are vital to the infant's future quality of life.

In the past 70 years public policy affecting disabled infants and children has been formulated at the local, state and federal level. Following the lead of

[*] Professor of Community Medicine and Director, Health Policy Program, School of Medicine, University of California, San Francisco.

[†] Pre-doctoral Fellow at the Health Policy Program, School of Medicine, University of California, San Francisco.

New York City and several states, the federal government
began its involvement with the health of women and children in 1912 with the establishment of the Children's
Bureau. During the 1920's it maintained a grant-in-aid
program to states in an effort to reduce infant and
maternal mortality. However, the program was voluntary
on the part of the states, and it was discontinued in
1929.

The Social Security Act in 1935 established not
only the present Social Security System, but also a
permanent program of grants-in-aid to the states to support maternal and child health and crippled children's
programs. This set the pattern of public assistance
payments that has persisted to this day. The federal
program supporting state Crippled Children's Services
followed by more than a decade the institution of such
programs in many states.

Since the early federal intervention in 1912, a
confusing variety of policies and programs for the disabled have come into being. Although not specifically
directed at infants with handicapping conditions, many
of the programs provide some resources or aid in their
medical care, financial support or rehabilitation.
Since it is not possible to discuss all these programs
in detail, our discussion is limited to five programs
particularly important to children who may require long
term care:

    1. Crippled Children's Services (CCS)
    2. Mental Retardation Services
    3. Special Educational Services
    4. Social and Rehabilitation Services
    5. Medicaid

CRIPPLED CHILDREN'S SERVICES

Many states began to develop programs in the 1920's
to serve the medical needs of crippled children. The
1935 enactment of Title V of the Social Security Act

provided federal grants to states for maternal and child
health services, services for crippled children and child
welfare services. Since that time, every state has developed its own program, usually financed with federal,
state, and local government funds. The objective is to
locate crippled children and to provide assistance with
diagnosis, treatment, and rehabilitation--including
hospitalization, surgical and corrective care when required. Children of many families that cannot pay for
medical care are enabled to obtain the services of the
appropriate specialists and institutions.

The original emphasis of Crippled Children's Services was on orthopedic problems and congenital malformations. Later the program gradually expanded to include a variety of other conditions. About one-fourth
of the children treated currently suffer from diseases
affecting the nervous system and the sense organs (cerebral palsy, epilepsy), another one-fourth have diseases of the bones, joints and muscles, and one-fifth
have congenital malformations (congenital heart disease, cleft palate).[1] Although the program has expanded,
children with birth defects still account for the largest
single group treated under the Crippled Children's
Services.[2]

MENTAL RETARDATION SERVICES

Until recently, the needs of the mentally retarded
have been ignored altogether or accorded a low priority
in federal programs. The burden was left to rest on
the families of the retarded, to charity, or to the state
governments that usually provided only custodial care.
It was not until the passage of the National Mental
Health Act in 1946 and the establishment of the National
Institute of Mental Health in 1949 that any federal role
in services for the mentally retarded was evident. In
1963, under the stimulus of President John F. Kennedy,
the federal government began to take a more serious interest in the problem.

The first significant federal aid for the mentally
retarded was authorized with the 1963 passage of the
Mental Retardation Facilities and Community Health Center Construction Act. The Mental Retardation amendments
of 1967 provided staffing grants and funds to expand and
upgrade residential care, and a variety of other programs with federal financial support in the 1960's offered some assistance to the mentally retarded.

Improvements in the programs of some states followed enactment in 1970 of the Developmental Disabilities
Services and Facilities Improvement Amendments. For example, outpatient clinics of varying degrees of compre-
hensiveness have been established in 44 states, the
District of Columbia, and Puerto Rico to serve the medical, psychological and social needs of the mentally
retarded. One-third of these clinics are in five states:
Washington, California, North Carolina, New Jersey, and
Virginia.[3] These clinics provided evaluation, treatment, and follow-up services to 57,000 children in 1971.
But this limited program does not begin to reach the
estimated 2.5 million mentally retarded under age 20.[4]

California has dealt with the fragmentation of
services by establishing an exemplary network of regional
centers. These provide comprehensive services and continuity of care to mentally retarded of all ages and
levels of disability. This system began with state
legislation in 1965 that created two pilot regional centers. In 1969 the program was expanded to provide centers in a number of cities well distributed geographi-
cally throughout the state. The centers make referrals
to appropriate agencies and provide services that are
not covered by other programs. Arrangements for placement in private or state institutions are also made
through the centers. Parents may reimburse the centers
according to their ability to pay.

Special Educational Services

Medical complications at birth may lead to mental
or learning disabilities that appear later. Until

recently, children with these problems had limited opportunities for education: public or private residential facilities, private schools, or public schools
without special assistance. Since 1972, however, court
decisions have laid the groundwork for guaranteeing
every child, disabled or not, a right to education within the public school system.[5] Schools are slowly moving
towards identifying, evaluating, and providing services
to all children with special needs. A variety of techniques, including special day classes, itinerant special
education teachers, and supplemental resources for the
normal classroom, are used in an effort to meet these
needs.

The federal government has had limited involvement
in special education. Of the $2.7 billion spent on
special education in 1971, only $315 million or 12 per-
cent were federal expenditures.[6] A number of loosely
related programs have developed, with a variety of functions. The primary emphasis of these federal programs
has been stimulation of state and local development and
the support of innovation within the field.

Social and Rehabilitation Services

Disabled children may be eligible for a wide range
of programs that fall into the category of "social services," including primarily cash benefits and social
services. Because of the large numbers of poor people
who receive assistance, social services expenditures
account for 50 percent of all federal, state and local
government spending.[7] These benefits are most often
provided to needy people who fall into one of the categories of public assistance, and to families with dependent children, the blind, the aged, and the disabled.

A recently added social service benefit is supplemental security income, under Title XVI of the Social
Security Act. Disabled persons who have a countable
income of less than $130 a month qualify after the age
of 18. They are eligible before age 18, but parental

income is considered in determining payments if the child lives at home. The minimum payment to those eligible is $146 a month. Many states supplement this amount with payments of their own, and provide automatic eligibility for Medicaid for those who qualify for supplementary security income payments.

Disabled persons who qualify for welfare are eligible for a variety of services such as day care, recreation, transportation assistance, and vocational rehabilitation. Such professional and paraprofessional services are supported by federal grants to the states. Rehabilitation programs have emphasized vocational rehabilitation. Medical and medically directed rehabilitation services may be provided if there is a reasonable expectation that the services will enable the handicapped individual to engage in a gainful occupation.

Medicaid

Medicaid is a state-federal program that finances medical services for the categorically needy and, in some states, for the medically needy. Those eligible under the categorical assistance programs (defined below) are families with dependent children who are receiving public assistance, and many aged, blind, and disabled persons eligible for supplementary income payments. One-half of the states also finance services for the medically needy, i.e., those persons who have incomes above the public assistance level, but who are unable to pay their medical expenses. Medicaid is often used as a supplement to or total payment for services provided crippled children, the mentally ill and disabled adults. The federal Office of Management and Budget has estimated that medical care services under Medicaid will be provided to approximately 26 million recipients in the fiscal year 1976. The federal outlays will be $7.2 billion and state and local governments will provide an additional $6.9 billion.[8]

WHERE POLICIES FAIL

The programs just described indicate that the government at every level has been willing to help provide for disabled children. Services are available. Federal, state, and local funds may be used either to pay for the services or provide them directly. Nevertheless, the value and effectiveness of these programs are impaired by fragmentation and poor coordination of services, uneven distribution of benefits and inadequate funding. Although individual programs may be adequate for their stated purposes, when viewed as a whole by parents, physicians, social workers and others concerned with disabled children, they appear as a jungle of diverse, complicated and sometimes contradictory eligibility, services, and payment provisions.

Fragmentation, the term that perhaps best characterizes the health services available for disabled children of poor or low income families, includes:

1. separation of preventive and curative services

2. separation of ambulatory from inpatient services

3. multiple financial or other eligibility requirements

4. difficult access to care and a need to make repeated reentries into the care system

5. substantial travel time to seek appropriate or specialized care

6. reliance on multiple sources of financing

7. services of uneven quality because of multiple regulatory standards

8. extravagant duplication of functions

9. isolation of health services from other
    essential community services

10. gaps in health service, and provision
    of care according to criteria based on
    age, income, residence, or kind of
    disease[9]

The same characteristics may be found in social
and educational services for the mentally retarded, and
in rehabilitation services for the disabled. Coordination of the full array of social, educational, and
medical services is seldom achieved.

Categories and Fragmentation

Most federal health programs are "categorical,"
that is, are allocated for specific populations or intended to deal with a specific problem. For example,
Crippled Children's Services was organized on a categorical model. Although this helps assure that the
needs of many of those with specific disabling illnesses
are not overlooked, others, whose problems are not so
easily categorized, may find it difficult to obtain
assistance.

A fragmented system poses great obstacles to effective coordination. Thus, the piecemeal categorical
approach results in a great number of agencies, each
with its own eligibility requirements, benefits, services and bureaucracy. Limited funds make each program
sensitive to the possible duplication of services and
reluctant to assume expenditures that another program
might pay for. Large administrative bureaucracies
evolve to assure that applicants have made every effort
to acquire help from all other possible sources. Robert
Morris, Professor of Social Planning at Brandeis University, has these comments on social services and the
effect of the categorical approach:

> Present categories of service are
> often designed to turn applicants
> away rather than help them. There
> is a low probability that anyone
> actively seeking help will actually
> get any help and even less probabil-
> ity that the help received will be
> geared to that applicant's life plan.[10]

Distribution and Priorities

Uneven distribution of benefits is another major
problem with federally supported programs for the disabled. Services are arbitrarily and inequitably rationed
among those who succeed in overcoming such access barriers as differences in availability of services according to the handicap and state involved, great variations in expenditures, need to travel long distances,
or need to queue for services.

Differing priorities among states have caused
marked differences among programs. In the Crippled
Children's Services, for example, states vary greatly
in their coverage of disease categories. Thus, a child
with a particular problem may receive extensive benefits
in one state while one with the same condition may receive little or no assistance in another state.[11]

Uneven distribution of benefits is evident in the
great differences in expenditures between states, and
even within large states. In 1970, Medicaid payments
per child recipient averaged only $43 in Mississippi,
but were $133 in New York. Moreover, only one-tenth
of the poor children in Mississippi received Medicaid
benefits, while nearly all the poor and near poor children in New York received them.[12]

Coverage may also be limited because of the location
of services and necessary queuing. For example, a
Connecticut study revealed that children attending five
Crippled Children's Services clinics came almost en-
tirely from areas immediately around the clinics.[13]

The waiting time to place a retarded child in an institution can be as long as five months in California, and
even longer in many other states. Meanwhile, parents
may be wholly unable to obtain the necessary service
without the financial and social assistance of the appropriate public agency.

Added to these problems is restricted funding.
Programs for the needy have always been kept close to
minimal levels in relation to needs. Federal expenditures for children's health care have also been con-
sistently low in Crippled Children's Services, special
education, Medicaid and other programs designed to help
meet their needs.

Inadequate funding means that not all who are eligible will benefit. Only 59 percent of all handicapped
youth between the ages of 5-17 have access to necessary
special education[14] while millions of poor children
have inadequate access to needed health care services.
In Connecticut, one of the nation's wealthiest states,
it is estimated that only one-half of the children who
need Crippled Children's Services receive such care.[15]

CONCLUSION

We have outlined many problems with current medical
and social programs for disabled children. Participants
involved in decisionmaking within a neonatal intensive
care unit must be aware of these programs, and of their
many inadequacies. This is not to suggest that decisions hinge on estimates of the child's future treatment
within the tangle of social welfare and health programs.
But ignorance of the programs and their difficulties
may deny a child services that could be beneficial, or
create unrealistic expectations that will have serious
adverse effects on the child and the family. The need
for reevaluation of programs and reform is increasingly
apparent.

Undoubtedly the choice will often be to sustain
the life of an individual who may later need help from

these services despite program inadequacies and difficulties of providing or paying for long term care. Our
responsibility is to propose and promote the program
changes needed to assure the best opportunity for each
infant who may survive initial neonatal intensive care
with a chronic disability.

Ethical Issues in Neonatal Intensive Care:
An Economic Perspective

Marcia J. Kramer[*]

Neonatal Intensive Care (NIC) has revolutionized the practice of pediatric medicine in recent years, and in the process it has effected sharp reductions in infant mortality rates. As is so often the case, however, progress has proven to be a mixed blessing. Because of the high incidence of congenital anomalies and extreme prematurity among the NIC population, a disproportionate share of those saved by early treatment die later in childhood or suffer severe and permanent impairment. From this most tragic circumstance springs the ethical dilemma at the heart of the present essay: Is it ever morally right to withhold NIC from a baby whose life depends on it?

In recognition of the fact that NIC is an economic good--even as it is a moral (or immoral) endeavor--this paper views the ethics of the treatment decision from an economic perspective. The first section examines the relevance of cost considerations to the formulation of a moral NIC policy, and then explores the appropriateness of technical economic solutions. The conceptual

---

[*]
Assistant Professor of Economics, Health Sciences Center, State University of New York, Stony Brook.

problems encountered in measuring the cost of NIC are
discussed in the second section. Data on hospitalization
costs at the Medical Center of the University of California at San Francisco serve to illustrate many of the
points raised.

THE RELEVANCE OF ECONOMICS

The readiness of economists to address an ever wider
range of decision problems in cost-benefit terms has
suffused the professional literature with new and valuable insights.[1] However, this willingness to tackle
problems outside their traditional areas of competence
may not impress others as being sufficient justification
for the intrusion of efficiency experts into the realm
of ethics. Rather than merely assuming the relevance
of economics to a resolution of the ethical issues raised
by neonatal intensive care, this matter is considered
explicitly at the outset.

Cost as a Factor

Is it ever right to deny neonatal intensive care
on the grounds of excessive cost? For an economist,
this question is pivotal. If the answer is "no", then
all facts pertaining to the economic implications of
NIC--no matter how important to parents, hospital admin-
istrators, and insurers--are simply irrelevant to the
ethical dilemma of whether or not to treat.

While moral questions are not those that public
opinion can definitively resolve, it should be recognized
that there is considerable resistance to the establishment of most criteria for NIC.[2] Two arguments are offered in support of the costs-are-irrelevant position:

(1) In its essentials, the problem confronting us
is not economic. If an infant's medical condition is
so poor that there is a high probability of severe impairment should he survive intensive care, the morality

of providing it is questionable even if the cost of so doing is zero. It follows that economic factors should play no part in our resolution of the problem.

(2) NIC is vital to human life, and human life is more valuable than anything that money can buy. But the "right to life" is no right at all if a helpless individual is denied the means necessary to preserve his life. NIC must therefore be regarded as a basic human right. Certainly the child who, with medical help, can be expected to lead a reasonably normal existence should not be denied survival because of costs. Because they reflect moral absolutes, questions of right and wrong can never be adequately answered in terms of mere dollars and cents.

Evaluating the Arguments

Though superficially persuasive, each of these arguments collapses upon close examination. In answer to the first, it is of course true that cost may not be responsible for creating the ethical dilemma, but inevitably it does add another dimension to the problem. If a physician were to treat cancer without regard for the probable adverse side effects of his drugs, the "cure" might well be more devastating than the disease. If the debate on NIC is to be more than academic, and the ethical positions espoused are to be fit for implementation in the real world, then it is imperative that policy be formulated with a view to its probable repercussions.

The second argument, humanitarian though it may seem, becomes increasingly weaker as it is carried to its logical extreme. Eventually, the moral principle that life should be sustained at any cost becomes inconsistent as the *real* cost of employing scarce resources to keep a particular person alive is measurable in terms of other lives. We need not look far beyond the boundaries of our affluent society to find the alternatives presented in such stark form. The chronic scarcity of

medical manpower and facilities in the developing nations
is such that a diversion of these resources to NIC would
almost certainly jeopardize the lives of other would-be
patients.[3] Even if sufficient resources could be transferred out of other economic activities and into the
medical sector, the fact that fertility and infant mortality rates are both so very high in these countries
means that NIC hospitalization costs alone could easily
reduce per capita income to a level incompatible with
life.[4]

If other lives are not at stake, there is no in-
consistency inherent in the argument that NIC should
take precedence over all other economic goods and services. However, it is hard to appreciate the morality
of a rule so utterly unconcerned with the quality of
life that it would sooner reduce everyone to a subsis-
tence standard rather than deny care to a single, ailing
newborn, for whom the odds may not be favorable. A
universally applicable NIC policy that aspires to morality *must* provide for drawing the line on costs. As philosophy professor Charles Frankel has observed, every
principle has its slippery slope: The "sanctity of
human life" does not everywhere dominate the "duty to
use limited human resources discriminatingly."[5]

Problems of a Market Mechanism

It is one thing to acknowledge the relevance of
economic considerations to a resolution of the ethical
dilemma posed by NIC, but quite another to determine
just where the line should be drawn. What guidance
can technical economic analysis offer with regard to
this critical issue?

The allocation of most goods and services in our
economy is determined by the functioning of the price
system. In the absence of market imperfections, this
system insures that the consumers of a product are
those and only those persons who are willing and able
to pay a price sufficient to cover the marginal costs

of its production. If all individuals, acting rationally, spend their incomes on the items that yield them a maximum of benefit per dollar cost, a situation results in which no one can be made better off without someone else being made worse off (economists call this "Pareto optimality" or "economic efficiency"). Few ethicists could quarrel with the desirability of this state; surely it would be wrong to prevent someone from reaching an attainable consumption goal if no one else would be disadvantaged in the process.

The question naturally arises whether the market mechanism can be relied upon to provide a morally acceptable solution to the NIC dilemma. To this, the answer is a definitive "no". In terms of economic efficiency, the forces of supply and demand would produce a sub-optimal solution owing to the presence of (1) consumption externalities (i.e. not all benefits accrue to the parents, who are the consumers, nor are all the costs incurred by them); (2) decreasing marginal costs of production (i.e. except in fully utilized facilities, marginal cost pricing cannot cover the high fixed costs of equipping and staffing an NIC unit for round-the-clock duty); and (3) unusually difficult financing problems (i.e. without catastrophic insurance coverage very few people who would have willingly insured against this risk could afford to pay the full cost associated with NIC; yet with such coverage there is a danger of overutilization because price fails to act as a constraint). In terms of equity, the market solution is more objectionable still, at least to an egalitarian, since children of the poor would be effectively excluded from the life-saving treatment that might be available to other children.

Cost-Benefit Analysis as a Solution

The inadequacy of a laissez-faire NIC policy does not preclude other technical economic solutions. Increasingly, economists have been promoting cost-benefit

analysis on a societal (as opposed to individual) scale
when, for reasons of equity and/or efficiency, market
solutions are deemed inappropriate. At least one economist has already urged application of the cost-benefit
approach to the problem of decisions on NIC treatment.[6]
In effect, the cost-benefit method attempts to correct
for all of the imperfections in the market test rule
while keeping intact the principle of consumer sover-
eignty. If, after these corrections, the combined amount
that all members of society would be willing to spend on
NIC for a particular child exceeds the expected cost of
a positive decision, then, by this rule, care should be
given. Otherwise, care should be withheld.

Certainly, it would be wonderful if the reasonably
objective cost-benefit method could generate morally
correct answers to the recurrent dilemma of whether or
not to give NIC. Regrettably, it is wholly inadequate
to this task because it operates without reference to
any moral principles. It requires only that social welfare be maximized. For a society composed of morally
upright individuals, cost-benefit analysis would produce
a moral solution. For a society that happens to be
peopled with immoral persons who--for whatever reasons
of their own--feel that the death of some or all babies
(even healthy ones) would enhance their welfare, or
further their goals, cost-benefit analysis may yield
an immoral solution. Implicit in the method is the assumption that the worth of a baby, like the worth of
any other consumer good, is identically equal to the
benefits that baby is capable of providing *to others*,
and that the fact of its existence in and of itself entitles the child to no claim on life. Unless external
constraints can somehow be incorporated into the cost-
benefit method, there is no assurance that its solution
will be ethical, as well as "optimal."

THE ECONOMIC IMPLICATIONS OF
NEONATAL INTENSIVE CARE

Although the tools of economic analysis are ill
suited to the task of ethical decisionmaking, the

economic implications of decisions are perfectly legitimate considerations in the formulation of moral policies.
This section is therefore devoted to a discussion of the
economics of NIC.

What costs are incurred by a decision to provide
NIC? The question is straightforward, and yet the answer depends in great part on the ethical framework of
the policy maker.

Cost and Duration of Commitment

The first issue is the duration of the commitment
implied by a decision to give NIC. If it is considered
perfectly moral to review this decision periodically as
the child's course progresses, then only those costs to
be incurred prior to the next reappraisal are relevant
to the treatment decision at the time. For example, if
it is understood that an initial decision to actively
support life may by good conscience be reversed at a
later point in the child's hospital stay when the prognosis is much more certain, then only the immediate
medical care costs of NIC should be considered as a potential deterrent to a positive first decision.

Of course, this notion that treatment might be instituted without any long-term commitment to the child's
survival is not likely to find many adherents even among
those who could support a denial of care under certain
conditions at the time of birth. If morality dictates
that the decision to provide NIC constitutes a commitment
on the part of society to meet the needs of the patient-
individual until such time as he can be self-sufficient,
then a much longer view of costs is required.

Data from the Medical Center of the University of
California at San Francisco indicate the magnitude of
the neonatal medical care costs that are necessarily incurred by an initial decision to treat. For eight children with birth weights under 1200 grams, hospitalization
bills in 1973 averaged $9,586 (Table 1). The much lower

Table 1

COSTS OF HOSPITALIZATION FOR 60 INFANTS RECEIVING INTENSIVE CARE,
BY CONDITION AT BIRTH AND BY OUTCOME
UCSF, 1969-73

| | Respiratory Distress Syndrome(a) June 1969-Dec. 1970 | Birth Weight Less Than 1500 Grams(b) | | | |
| | | 1969 | | 1973 | |
		Less than 1200 grams	1200-1500 grams	Less than 1200 grams	1200-1500 grams
Cost Per Patient(c)	$ 4,768	$ 6,597	$ 5,218	$ 9,586	$12,351
Died	3,144	2,600	4,071	3,885	1,071
Normal	4,768	-	5,600	26,690	13,761
Abnormal	23,836	14,590	-	-	-
No. Days Per Patient	29.0	38.0	51.1	27.4	39.9
Died	13.9	9.5	30.0	7.0	2.0
Normal	30.4	-	58.2	88.5	44.6
Abnormal	116.0	95.0	-	-	-
Cost Per Patient Day	$ 165	$ 174	$ 102	$ 350	$ 310
Died	227	273	136	555	535
Normal	148	-	96	302	308
Abnormal	205	154	-	-	-
Cost Per Survivor	$ 6,357	$19,791	$ 6,957	$38,344	$13,894
Number of Patients	32	3	8	8	9
Died	8	2	2	6	1
Normal	23	0	6	2	8
Abnormal	1	1	0	0	0

(a) Sample, patients born at or transferred to UCSF.

(b) All infants born at UCSF.

(c) Cost per patient is obtained by dividing total costs incurred by patients in each category by the total number of patients in that category. Cost per survivor is obtained by dividing total costs for all patients (regardless of outcome) by the number of survivors.

in-hospital death rate (and consequent lengthier hospital stay) of the nine babies in the 1200-1500-gram category accounts for their appreciably higher average bill of $12,351. On a per diem basis, average costs were in fact less for this relatively healthy group, $310 as opposed to $350. Though the sample is small, the data on children treated for respiratory distress syndrome in 1969-70 and born with low weights in 1969 demonstrate the much greater level of hospitalization costs among abnormal survivors of NIC than among their normal counterparts.

To the uninsured couple contemplating NIC for their offspring, the variability in hospitalization costs may be of greater concern than the mean figure, substantial though it is: In five of these 17 low birth weight cases observed in 1973, the bill exceeded $18,000, and in two instances it was greater than $28,000. Despite reductions in average length of stay, total cost per patient evidenced a sharp upward trend over the period 1969-1973, rising 45 percent for the less than 1200-gram group and 137 percent for the 1200-1500-gram group. These increases reflect the doubling and tripling of cost per day in the two groups, respectively. Should the totals continue to grow at these rates, many persons who now dismiss NIC costs as irrelevant or inconsequential are likely to reconsider their opinions in the near future.

Costs and Outcomes

If long-term costs are indeed mandated by NIC, their nature would depend upon the outcome of care. Because NIC yields the consumer a set of medically indicated procedures rather than a guaranteed result, outcomes are not predictable with certainty. The *infant who dies* while in the hospital clearly incurs no cost beyond that of intensive care itself.

For the *normal survivor* of NIC, post-neonatal costs are similar to those of any healthy newborn. In the

early years, there are direct and indirect costs of
childrearing, the former including such things as food,
clothing and educational expenses, and the latter principally consisting of the mother's foregone earnings.
U.S. data show that the (undiscounted) cost of raising
a first child through college graduation totaled $98,361
in 1969 for the moderate-income family.[7] After maturity,
the expenditure flow typically reverses as the average
individual generates income in excess of his personal
consumption.[8]

By comparison, for *the severely abnormal survivor*
of NIC, the long term cost picture is decidedly negative.
To normal consumption expenditures must be added the
costs of institutionalized custodial care (or additional
foregone earnings if the child is cared for by a parent
at home), special education, and extraordinary medical
expenses. Instead of there being an eventual offset to
childhood costs, the total continually mounts if the
individual's productivity never suffices to cover his
ordinary consumption requirements.

Assuming that public institutions for the mentally
retarded are representative in this respect, custodial
care costs alone averaged $3,450 per patient per year
in 1970. An additional $2,500 per annum was expended
for each institutionalized child under 20 to cover educational and other developmental activities. "Normal"
consumption for the institutionalized population was
then $1,173 per resident per year.[9] Thus, even if long-
term care is given in institutions hardly known for
their extravagance, the financial cost to society of an
economically unproductive individual who requires a
full lifetime of institutionalized care is likely to
exceed $400,000.[10]

Costs and Quality of
Continued Care

This points to a second critical assumption that
influences the costing of NIC. Specifically, what

"quality of life" is envisioned for the post-neonatal period? The dollar costs associated with NIC are relatively low if society makes only minimal provisions for its handicapped members, but if society strives to offer a superior level of care to those in need, NIC is likely to be much more expensive. It is illustrative in this regard to note that in 1970 the average yearly cost of care per patient was $6,640 in public mental hospitals as against $23,067 in private mental hospitals.[11]

Alternatives to NIC

There is yet a third way in which ethical judgments on the part of society condition the measurement of the aggregate NIC cost. To be meaningful, the cost incurred by a decision to purchase X must be stated net of any costs that would be incurred by a decision not to purchase X. With most goods and services, the cost of not purchasing is simply zero, and the distinction between total and incremental costs is empty.

A decision to withhold NIC, however, is not necessarily costless. If the alternative to intensive care is mercy killing, then the assumption of a zero-cost basis is valid. If ordinary, non-heroic measures are undertaken to sustain infants denied intensive care, however, this assumption is not generally warranted, because some babies eligible for NIC can usually be expected to survive without it. Where severe impairment is the probable outcome for such would-be survivors, the comparison cost of *not* administering special medical treatment in infancy may be substantial. It is thus possible that even if provision of NIC for certain infants were judged very costly vis-à-vis an active policy of euthanasia, such care would yield real cost-savings to communities that otherwise would have allowed nature to take its course with ailing newborns.[12]

In view of the above considerations, and given the uncertainty of outcomes in individual cases, the expected dollar cost associated with a decision to provide NIC to a baby with a particular medical condition is:

$$(1) \quad E = \sum_{i=1}^{3} P_{it}(N_i + C_{it} - B_i) - \sum_{i=1}^{3} P_{iw}(C_{iw} - B_i),$$

where:

E = expected net incremental dollar cost incurred by providing NIC.

N_i = the medical care cost of NIC itself for a child with eventual outcome i (usually $N_3 > N_2 > N_1$);

C_{it} = other direct and indirect dollar costs incurred during the lifetime of a child who is given intensive care at birth (t = treated) and whose eventual outcome is i (usually $C_3 > C_2 > C_1$);

C_{iw} = direct and indirect dollar costs incurred during the lifetime of a child who is denied intensive care (w = treatment withheld) and whose eventual outcome is i ($C_{1w} = 0$ if euthanasia is the alternative to care, $C_{iw} = C_{it}$ otherwise);

B_i = dollar benefits yielded over the lifetime of a child with eventual outcome i ($B_2 > B_3 > B_1 = 0$);

i = 1: an infant death
i = 2: a normal survivor
i = 3: an abnormal survivor

P_{it}, P_{iw} = probability of outcome i given treatment decision t or w, respectively, where

$$\sum_{i=1}^{3} P_{it} = \sum_{i=1}^{3} P_{iw} = 1$$

The Formula and A Hypothetical Example

A hypothetical example can best illustrate exactly how the various factors interact to determine expected cost through this formula. Consider a medical condition for which NIC would drastically lower the probability of death occurring in infancy (p_1 falling from .8 without care to .1 with it), but where few of those saved would be capable of leading a normal life (p_2 rising from .1 to .2, but p_3 rising from .1 to .7). Assume that the cost of the intensive care necessary for achieving this change in the outcome probabilities averages $15,000 for each abnormal survivor, $10,000 per normal survivor, and $5,000 per infant death (cost being an increasing function of length-of-hospital-stay and extent of disability).

Further assume that the net cost, exclusive of neonatal medical care expenses that the children in question impose on society (i.e., the excess of the value of their consumption over their production) is close to zero for those who die in infancy; negative for normal survivors (i.e., they constitute a net benefit); and very high for abnormal survivors [say, $C_1 - B_1$) = $400, ($C_2 - B_2$)= -$50,000, and ($C_3 - B_3$) = $300,000].[13] It follows that the expected incremental cost of providing NIC for a baby born with this condition is $187,720: Expected cost with care [.10 ($5,000 + $400) + .20 ($10,000 - $50,000) + .70 ($15,000 + $300,000)] minus expected cost without care [.80 ($400) + .10 (-$50,000) + .10 ($300,000)] = $187,720.

Contrast this now with a situation in which NIC brings about only a small reduction in infant mortality but vastly improves the prospects for those who survive (say, p_{1w} = .15, p_{2w} = .05, and p_{3w} = .80, with the p_{it} all as before). With no change in the N_i, C_i, or B_i, the expected incremental cost of providing NIC would here be -$24,520 per child. On purely financial grounds, a policy of treatment would in this case be socially advantageous. If abnormal outcomes were costlier still [say, ($C_3 - B_3$) = $385,400], E might range from as high as $400,000 (if p_{1w} = p_{3t} = 1.0) to as low as -$425,000 (if p_{3w} = p_{2t} = 1). Clearly, the cost of providing NIC may vary enormously from one condition to the next, even if medical care costs per se are approximately the same.

Who might use a formula such as (1)? It is obvious
that neither parents nor hospitals are likely to view
the financial implications of NIC in these terms; particularly since so many of the component cost and benefit
items in E are external to each of these parties. And
yet, it must be emphasized that the full social cost
(or benefit) of NIC is an economic reality, even if treatment decisions are not now predicated upon it. Since
the interests of *all* affected parties deserve consideration in the formulation of an NIC *policy*, it is incum-
bent upon those involved in the formulation of such
policies to view at some point the cost problem from a
societal perspective.

ADDITIONAL ECONOMIC CONSIDERATIONS

The economic input into the formulation of a moral
NIC policy should properly encompass more than a dollar
measure of the expected total cost of providing care.
Of equal importance is information concerning the incidence of this net incremental cost, both inter-generationally and cross-sectionally (i.e. among diverse individuals), and the probable effectiveness of treatment.

Temporal Dimension of NIC Costs

The incremental dollar costs and benefits associated
with a decision to provide NIC are realized over a period
of many years, often decades. If cost cut-offs are to
be established, it is necessary that the stream of annual net incremental costs be collapsed into a single
summary figure. To do this, a rate of time preference
must be specified so that costs incurred in different
years can be transformed into like units. For reasons
of simplicity, equation (1) implicitly assumed a zero
discount rate (i.e., the C_S and B_S are simple summations
of annual C_S and B_S, respectively). In contrast, the
standard practice of economists is to adopt a positive
rate of discount.

Since it is our express purpose here to identify economic factors relevant to the formulation of a *moral* policy, the moral implications of this discounting practice warrant explicit consideration. A positive discount rate assigns a weight to each year's expected net incremental cost (benefit) which diminishes with the length of time elapsing between the present and given year. From the viewpoint of society as constituted at time t, it is no doubt correct to assume that gains realizable in the immediate future are valued more highly than those not realizable for many years hence.

Whether it is morally right to use a decision rule that gives preference to the present as against future generations, is another matter. The effect of such a rule is to make it relatively difficult to justify NIC on cost grounds for the would-be normal child requiring moderately high neonatal medical care expenditures, while making it relatively easy to justify such care for the would-be abnormal child whose immediate medical needs are much more modest.[14]

Inter-Personal Dimension of NIC Costs

The distribution of net incremental costs and benefits must be acceptable cross-sectionally as well as inter-temporally if an affirmative NIC decision is to be morally correct. UCSF data for 1969-1970 indicate that NIC hospitalization costs are borne primarily by society at large (i.e., by taxpayers, health insurers, and all hospital patients) rather than by the families of children in the intensive care unit. Thus, patient families were the single most important source of financing in only 5.1 percent of the 59 cases sampled, and direct patient payments accounted for only 2.4 percent of total hospital charges (Table 2). The long term care picture likewise indicates a preponderance of publicly assumed costs, with only 13.6 percent of institutional expenditures for the mentally retarded being made in private facilities in 1970.[15]

Table 2

HOSPITALIZATION COSTS FOR 59 INFANTS
TREATED FOR RESPIRATORY DISTRESS
SYNDROME BY SOURCE OF PAYMENT
UCSF, JUNE 1969-DECEMBER 1970

Total cost: $259,144

Cost per patient: 4, 329

Distribution of total costs
  by source of payment:

Patient	2.4%
Insurance	42.8
Medi-Cal	15.2
Hospital budget	29.6
Private grants	6.7
County funds	1.0
Crippled Children's Society	2.3
TOTAL	100.0%

Distribution of patients
  by primary source of
  financing:

Patient	5.1%
Insurance	40.7
Medi-Cal	11.9
Hospital budget	33.9
Private grants	5.1
County funds	1.7
Crippled Children's Society	1.7
TOTAL (rounded)	100.0%

The fact that our affluent society at large bears
so much of the immediate and long-run monetary cost
associated with NIC has two implications for moral policy.
First, because the financial burden on any one family
is much less than it would be without such cost-sharing,
decisionmakers should be more inclined to regard any
given level of total net incremental cost as an acceptable price to pay. Second, in accordance with the principle of no taxation without representation, justice
would be served if society were given some voice in the
ultimate decision, since it does finally foot the bill.

Cost Effectiveness of NIC

Finally, effectiveness measures are needed if cost
data are to be seen in proper perspective. Even though
economics cannot tell us where we *should* draw the line
on costs, almost every one would agree that an expected
net incremental cost of, say, $25,000 per child treated
is more readily justifiable if 98 percent of the group
is expected to be normal following care than if 70 percent are expected to die in infancy and the remaining
30 percent are expected to be severely impaired, treatment notwithstanding.

In order to arrive at comparable cost figures for
infants with disparate prognoses at birth, it may be
helpful to think in terms of cost per successful outcome, however defined. If, for example, only normal
children were thought to have any moral worth, the expected NIC hospitalization cost per successful outcome
in 1973 would have been $38,344 for those in the less
than 1200-1500-gram group (Table 1). Alternately, if
one felt the identical moral obligation to treat all
babies in need, regardless of the probable outcome, then
the relevant comparison would be between total cost per
patient ($9,586 versus $12,351). By the latter standard,
the lower birthweight group would be more likely to
qualify for care if a cost-cutoff were established[16];
by the former, treatment of the higher birthweight group
would be deemed more cost effective.

SUMMARY

Neonatal intensive care resembles other economic goods and services in that its production necessitates the diversion of scarce resources from alternative uses. Because the activities foregone by providing NIC may be of greater moral worth than the care itself, it is morally imperative that cost criteria be established for this as for any other service. This is true regardless of the fact that NIC is often vital to human life.

Consumption externalities, decreasing marginal costs of production, and insurance coverage each interfere with the ability of the market mechanism to yield a Pareto-optimal (i.e. economically efficient) solution to the NIC problem. Cost-benefit analysis can surmount these technical difficulties, but it, too, presupposes the supremacy of consumer demands. Unless morality happens to be imbedded in the preference structure, there is no assurance that this alternate allocation rule will generate ethical solutions to the treatment dilemma.

Ethical problems arise both in the determination of moral cost ceilings, and in the measurement of cost. Thus, in order to evaluate the net dollar amount that will be incurred by a decision to provide NIC, one must first specify the duration of the commitment implied by treatment, the quality of long term care anticipated for the post-neonatal period, and the alternative to NIC. Depending upon the assumptions made and the medical condition at birth, average dollar cost per baby treated may range from something less than zero (i.e., a cost savings) to well in excess of $400,000.

In reaching a final decision, expected cost per patient is not the only economic factor to consider. Because rates of survival and permanent disability vary greatly from one condition to the next, decisions as to which medical conditions merit treatment should also focus on expected cost per successful outcome (however defined). In 1973, NIC hospitalization costs for babies under 1200 grams at birth averaged $9,586 at UCSF, yet as a result of high in-hospital mortality a total of $38,344 in hospital costs was expended per survivor. Finally, the incidence of costs must be acceptable both inter-generationally and cross-sectionally if a decision to provide NIC is to be morally correct.

In sum, though technical economic formulas can hardly be expected to resolve the moral problems posed by neonatal intensive care, economic considerations are highly pertinent to the ethical dilemma, and the economic framework of analysis provides a useful tool for systematically examining the consequences of treatment decisions on a case-by-case basis.

PART III

Questions of Policy

Having described the clinical reality and the social context of neonatal intensive care, we are now able to focus on questions of policy: decisions about norms and guidelines affecting neonatal intensive care.

F. Raymond Marks presents a framework for viewing the task of policy formation by drawing on relevant legal conceptions and certain implications of the Supreme Court decision on abortion. Michael Garland draws together the views of several professional ethicists--philosophers and theologians--who have written recently about the moral justifications and prohibitions of infant euthanasia. Finally, the essay by Albert Jonsen and Garland proposes a moral policy for neonatal intensive care. This essay focuses primarily on the more intimate questions of the clinical scene and the possibilities of parental involvement in decisions to continue treatment or to let death come. Without attempting a full elaboration of the problems, the essay also touches upon the larger policy issues of allocation of facilities and coordination of research.

The Defective Newborn: An Analytic Framework for a Policy Dialog

F. Raymond Marks*

(with the assistance of Lisa Salkovitz)[†]

INTRODUCTION

The development of neonatal intensive care units has led to the saving of many infant lives, lives that would have been terminated by nature had these units not existed. These units have also posed a series of dilemmas. Many of the children spared are normal and lead normal lives, but many others who are saved have defects sufficiently serious to make it highly unlikely that they will ever lead normal lives, and some will live lives that are hardly recognizable as human.

Thus biological and social viability have become further separated, emphasizing several questions: Should we try to save children when their prognosis is for a substandard human existence? Can other decisions be made using life-saving technological capabilities now available? Should defective lives be taken?

* Attorney, Childhood and Government Project, Boalt Hall, University of California, Berkeley.

[†]Research associate, Childhood and Government Project.

The authors are trained in law; while the paper contains a modicum of "legal" guidelines, the perspectives reflected are principally non-legal ones obtained by asking questions about how children are defined, viewed, treated and related to by society.

Newborn intensive care units raise three basic questions about childhood:

1. What is a child?

2. Who speaks for a child?

3. Who decides for a child?

The first question is directly posed by the issues this paper addresses. So far the dialog calls this cluster of issues "the quality of life." We suggest that *all* views of children--defective or so-called normal--involve "quality of life" questions. Society, the state, and parents define children less in terms of their "innate" nature, than in terms of what we want them to be in relation to society and the family. A child is both a biological creature and a social invention.

Questions of voice and decisionmaking, too, involve the same elements, particularly for neonates. A newborn child enjoys only a status relationship. He or she is dependent, totally dependent. Children are the creatures of society or their parents. This is true at least until they develop a voice, a will, a personality, and possess autonomy. The timing of children's independence is also a matter of social convention and convenience far more than it is a matter of biological development. By the time children reach maturity-- whether they be normal or defective--social choice, social agreement and social projection will have played a far larger role in what they have become than will their own intrinsic biological capacities or characteristics.

While the state and others play increasingly greater roles in the choices that are made for children, the family--the parents--remain the principal agency for determining what a child is or will be. Parents choose the child's religion, the form of his nurturing, the universe of his associations and much of the content of his life. Parents, in short, choose *what* a child will be. And, now, after the abortion decision--*Roe v. Wade*[1]--they even choose *whether* a child will be. The impact of this observation on the subject of this paper is obvious: The opportunities for ego projection are evident and the effects are nearly total.

This does not mean that a child does not have an existence--a being--separate from its parents, or that we do not have an interest in seeing or maintaining the separate reality of children. It means only that the neonatology decisions are but a small part of a persistent truth. As things now stand society and parents make most of the choices about what a child will be.

The subject we are examining, therefore, has a broader context that cannot be ignored. While it may be more dramatic, the on-the-spot decision to resuscitate a child is not too distant from many other daily decisions that will be made in the life of that child if it survives. Similarly, the social and abstract decision to allocate funds and energies to intensive care units, to maximize the survival chances of high risk infants, is not too distant from the decisions that society makes about allocating resources for the education of our children. As an examination of dependency and neglect cases would show, and as Jonathan Kozol's book[2] suggests, the survivors of childbirth can be killed many times over in their minds and their spirits. This larger context, too, cannot be ignored. If "success" in the intensive care units is unmatched by success elsewhere, biologically viable children may be unwanted children or uncared for children when they leave the nursery. For the clinician, this means that he should be more relaxed; he is not the majordomo of the only moments of truth in the lives of children.

What follows is an examination of the many facets of decisions that the medical profession, society, and parents are faced with as a result of the emerging ability to sustain life where previously it could not be sustained. The writers approach the task without commitment to particular decisions, and with considerable trepidation about the implications of some of our observations. We are convinced in a basic way, however, that the question before us is: "What decisions cannot be avoided?" And, because we are convinced that decisions will have to be made, much of this paper seeks to identify the actors, the interests of the actors and their capacity to make meaningful decisions.

A cautionary note: We, the writers, are abysmally ignorant of the state of the medical art. We have perhaps assumed too much from the literature, or too little. Where decisions require a high degree of medical certainty that does not now exist, we hope that we have not been too cavalier, and that we have fully spelled out our assumptions. In the last analysis, however, this caution does not slow us, because we are convinced that most of the decisions here are not medical decisions in a strict sense, but rather decisions about social policy and ethics.

QUESTION I:

Is it possible to have a legal standard or a social policy for intensive care nurseries that rests on premises other than saving lives at all costs?

As stated at the outset of this paper, the mixed blessing of newborn intensive care inevitably raises questions both about withholding therapy and actively terminating the lives of defective infants.[3]

Until quite recently the legal response to these questions, at least formally, would have been negative. When considering an identified individual life, the law did not recognize the "quality of life" issue.

The stance is exemplified in a suit brought against a physician by a defective infant (through a guardian ad litem, i.e., a guardian appointed for purposes of the lawsuit alone, where interests may differ from those of parents or natural guardians) and the child's parents. It was claimed that an opportunity was not offered for a therapeutic abortion after the mother contracted rubella, i.e., the risks were not communicated to the parents by the physician.[4] The theories of wrongful birth for the plaintiff infant and immense psychological and economic costs for the plaintiff parents failed to win compensation. Another theory, "wrongful conception," appears in two cases involving children born out of wedlock. The results were ambiguous. One court found that the act of giving life could not be said to contain an element of compensable harm[5] and the other that an injury could indeed be annexed to conception itself.[6]

Competing Values

However, the several decisions upholding a woman's right to obtain an abortion, culminating in the United States Supreme Court decision in *Roe v. Wade*, noted above, changed the right to life ethic. Birth, per se, and life, per se, were no longer the only values sanctioned. *Roe* recognized that there were competing values. A child's right to life had to be balanced against the mother's right of choice, the mother's right to life, impact on the family of an unwanted child, and even the impact upon the child if it were born an unwanted child. Narrowly and specifically the United States Supreme Court held that in the first trimester neither the state nor the medical profession has an interest in the decision to carry a fetus to term. It is the woman's decision alone. In the second trimester the state's interest grows, as does the interest of the medical profession. The emergence of state and medical interest was not, however, stated by the Court in *Roe* in terms of assuring the birth of the fetus; it was put in terms of assuring the safety and well being of the expectant mother. Only in the third trimester is society seen as having an interest in the life of the fetus.

Roe v. Wade has important implications for the neonatology dilemma. No matter what else is said about it, *Roe* is a quality of life decision. It recognizes that not one but two life-taking decisions are possible: the life of the fetus is seen as distinct from the life of the mother and of the family. It recognizes that there is a balancing that cannot be reached by a simplistic approach. And it holds, in the narrow sense, that the woman is the actor who must do the balancing. The same issues are present in the decisions facing the intensive care team and parents in the neonatology nursery, with one important difference. The court in *Roe* gives us a clue as to this difference. It held that a fetus in the first two trimesters was not a person within the meaning of the Fourteenth Amendment or other constitutional protections; until this point even the unborn child had no recognizable interest. This allowed the fetus to be aborted without considering it a "life." Such ease in the use of a non-life fiction is presently unavailable in the case of defective neonates.

Examining a Fiction

It is important to examine the meaning of the fiction in *Roe v. Wade*. Like all fictions it obscures the reality of a rule change.[7] A close analysis of the *Roe* decision requires a view that in reality the life of the fetus is taken in exchange for "saving" the life of the mother and the life of the family. Individual lives are exchanged and society's interest in preserving the family is asserted. But the fiction of fetal non-personhood enables the court to say it is making a life-saving decision for a known individual and making a life-taking decision only for an abstracted human. We can still have the pretense that the society will not tolerate life-taking for known individuals, while we have the reality of a rule that allows this result.

We can have an operational rule that relates to the "quality of life" and an announced rule that asserts the simplicity of the value of "saving human life at all costs."

Present hospital practices, reflected in some of the literature,[8] may already incorporate elements of a fiction. We now "let go" of some babies notwithstanding rules against euthanasia and the immateriality of the active-passive dichotomy (discussed below). But we do not announce this to the world. Such practice allows the actors to hide from themselves the fact that they have changed or departed from the rule while announcing their strict adherence to the absolute rule of sanctity of life in all cases.[9] In this connection, it is interesting to note that in *Roe v. Wade*, Mr. Justice Blackmun speaking for the majority, adopts a historical view that the Hippocratic Oath itself was a manifesto, not an expression of an absolute standard of medical conduct from which there could be no departure.[10]

Decisions and Costs

Consider now the observed dichotomy between abstract life-taking and life-saving decisions and decisions made in the cases of identified individuals. We should note under the former category some examples of wholesale departure from the standard of life-saving at all costs. The fact is: *Society makes decisions not to save lives at all costs*. The planning decisions that we already make involve life-taking. Dollars spent in the neonatology nursery may represent dollars not spent and lives lost in another segment of the health services delivery system. Indeed, conversely, dollars not spent in the intensive care units of the nurseries are life-taking decisions. Research expenditures also involve trade-offs that can be reckoned in the short and long term as life-taking as well as life-saving decisions. The same is true of decisions made by society as a whole in the allocation of public dollars among the health, transportation, education and so-called defense enterprises. The saving of human life has economic and social costs, costs that society as a whole may be unwilling to bear in all instances. Frequently we can make exact projections of the number of lives that will be lost if we do not expend a certain number of dollars. Examples in the fields of highway safety or air safety are numerous.

Identifying a Specific Life

Until *Roe v. Wade*, however, while society may have been willing to save dollars at the expense of human lives, or even save face at the expense of human lives, we have been unwilling to have this equation haunt us where we knew the identity of the lives to be taken or saved.[11] Calabresi demonstrates the difference in comparing decisions on highway safety to those we make when a single man is trapped in a coal mine. In the latter case we may even be willing to risk other unnamed human lives and other scarce resources to save the known man, whereas in the former we need only some assurance that we do not know the names of those whole lives a given policy will sacrifice.[12]

The human condition necessarily makes us frail when we consider that we may be the actors who have to accept the responsibility for making life and death decisions about human beings whom we can identify. *Roe v. Wade* forces a reexamination for several reasons.

How different is the decision in the nursery from that of the pregnant woman? We suggest that there is a substantial similarity, and there are also some important differences. First, the similarities. An unwanted fetus and an "unwanted" defective baby can be seen as strikingly similar when viewed in terms of parental hardship--economic and psychological--sibling hardship, social cost and other similar factors. An unwanted fetus, indeed, may be more viable and less costly than an unwanted defective child. The statistical chances of being accepted and achieving adjustment may be greater.

Effects on Parents

In a recent article, John Fletcher suggested that parents of defective children are personally devastated by the happening.[13] He makes some observations consistent with the thesis we have outlined in the introduction: parents have expectations for and about their children. The children are a projection of what the parent wants. Defective children frustrate their expectation in a profound and total way. The parent loses the validation of the child. Fletcher stated:

> Parents, especially the middle class, expect more intimacy and perfection in their children. Thus, the appearance of a defective newborn is more self-devastating than in an earlier time, when a family needed many children, and when children were not so regarded as expressions of the selves of the parents.[14]

In a discussion of amniocentesis (the analysis of amniotic fluid for genetic defects), Marc Lappe reflected the same sentiments and observations:

> As expected, the values of health and intelligence which their largely middle class style embodied, raised their expectations for these same qualities in their children. More insidiously, however, the very health, intelligence and normality of their yet-to-be-born children became what many of these parents used to formulate their own sense of adequacy and success.[15]

Seen in this way, the defective child is more
"unwanted" than the unplanned child. Can we say that
because the child was born alive the balancing of
lives that is permitted in *Roe v. Wade*--mother for
child--is out of the question? Does not a failure to
consider the trade-off condemn the parents as surely
as the earlier refusal to consider abortion condemned
the mother? An interesting public policy corollary
can be observed in adoption law, where adopting parents
can opt to place a mentally deficient or mentally ill
child with the state within five years of adoption for
conditions that existed at the time of adoption, but
were not discovered until later.[16] The adoption is
thereby cancelled. A warranty of fitness appears to
be involved, or at least notions of mistake. This
option is not now presently available for natural parents. In part that is what we are debating.

The Persistent Dilemma

The similarities to and the differences from *Roe*
having been examined, we still appear to be on the
horns of a dilemma. The life-saving ethic prevails.
Whether it prevails as a matter of conscious social
policy is immaterial. The specialized teams assembled
in intensive care units are inclined to and are trained
to fight for biological viability. In the small world
of the intensive care units, the training tutored by
the working ethic seems to prevent "letting go." It
is hard to imagine it to be otherwise.

The dilemma comes into play when we consider the
probabilities that under this practice, as social and
legal institutions are now arranged, the decisions
made and not made in the newborn intensive care unit
condemn the parents to untold suffering and burdens.
Further, the decisions impose substantial burdens on
the state and the society at large. As in the abortion field, pre-*Roe*, the singular decision to save a
baby's life at all costs may involve life-taking decisions when we view the other actors. When it turns

out that the baby will not enjoy an existence that we
can consider human or an existence outside of institutions, the dilemma becomes more apparent, and the
search for the way out becomes more imperative.

We end this section where we started: the adoption of a standard other than a "life-saving at all
costs" ethic does not seem to be permitted under the
existing legal standards and under prevailing social
practices tutored by both the law and our ethical
framework. But on the other hand, the adoption of a
different standard seems inevitable. An examination
of the recent literature[17] would appear to indicate
that nobody can live under a "business as usual" approach. Not making any decisions now is seen as making
a decision. For the balance of this paper, we will be
assuming: (a) that it is desirable to resolve the
dilemma--to find alternatives to life at all costs--
and (b) that there are infants for whom we can be
reasonably certain that we can accurately predict the
outcomes.

QUESTION II:

*What options are available for escaping from the
dilemma?*

In this section we will identify some possible
options so that the readers can have them in mind before we consider the when, how, and who of specific
decisionmaking. There are two major approaches to
solution: macro and micro. They overlap. But, essentially a macro-approach avoids the agony of specific decisionmaking that cannot be seen to have the
support of social agreement.

Consider the plight of the doctor who performed
"a therapeutic abortion" before the decision to abort
or not abort was considered to be the sole province
of the woman. The constituencies to whom the doctor
was accountable were diverse and unclear--the law,

his colleagues, the woman, and his conscience. Or,
consider the position of the doctor, now, who commits
an "act of mercy." The doctor is the sole decisionmaker. He is without social or collegial support, at
least not formally.

Macro-Decision Alternatives

Natural selection policy. At one extreme, if
society were unwilling to alter definitions of life and
death, and if it were unwilling to trust individual
decisionmaking that leads to the "taking" of some lives,
society could choose not to allocate present levels or
increased levels of resources and effort at the neonatology margins. Such a decision would be based on the
view that the benefit of saving many babies who turn
out to be normal is not great enough when reckoned in
terms of the cost of the increased increment of defective babies who are spared. This would be an option
of returning to an evolutionary course, abandoning
present intervention.

Rational selection policy. At the other extreme,
society could calculate that killing defective babies
would be the price paid for additional normal babies.
If so, it would accept the costs of redefining human
life to exclude the defective child. This would lead
to a redefinition of the law of murder--just as the
abortion decision leads to a redefinition of "life-
taking." This alternative presumes not only a willingness to construct an abstract definition of human viability in advance of the event of birth, but an ability
to define with enough particularity and consensus the
type of infant who, upon birth, would fit into the
category of "subhuman" non-personhood (infants with
spina bifida, i.e., divided spine; or extensive brain
damage). It also presumes a diagnostic ability that
may not at the moment exist.

The option is not altogether futuristic, although
it is dangerous. As a society, we have been able to

elect to spare lives at the cost of other lives, particularly where we are able to redefine the lives taken
as being "criminals," "enemies," or otherwise threatening. The legislative approach would be abstract, because it would be prospective in the same sense as the
abortion decision is prospective. We doubt that this
step will be taken, in the short-run, because it involves a major shift in our self-image.

   Welfare state policy. A possible intermediate
macro-approach would be to acknowledge the net benefit
of the normal babies spared, the extensive costs to
individual parents of defective children, and the enormous social costs of redefining life and murder. We
could then provide a mechanism for society to accept
the risk of defective children--allowing natural parents the same options that are now available to adop-
tive parents. Presently, even if a child is institutionalized, parents retain not only a psychological
responsibility, but a financial responsibility as well.
(Parents must contribute to the costs of institutionalized care.)[18]

   "Do nothing" policy. A fourth macro-decision
could be made--and it would be a decision--to do
nothing. This would be a decision to accept the dilemma created by the increased abilities to save
lives and the increasing amounts of resource allocation. There is a certain disingenuousness to this
decision, because it accepts as reality an assumption
that actors confronted with hard decisions do not
make decisions. The opposite is true: decisions are
now being made, but they are not policy-affecting decisions, because they are covert. A fiction is growing. Henry Dunlap, a hospital administrator, at the
Ross Conference[19] opted for this decision. He suggested that a common law of euthanasia would develop
(although he did not use these terms) in much the
same way that the common law of England had developed,
i.e.,by reacting to the actual decisions made in individual cases.

We do not agree. Individual decisions will not be reviewed, because they will not be discussed. As we have already indicated, a fiction will develop, actions will be taken by actors who will deny, even to themselves, that they are acting. To test the notion that fictions are developing one ought only to consider the language that has grown up around the intensive care units and around the emerging dialog about defective neonates. Considerable effort has been expended in attempting to distinguish between a passive posture, where the baby is allowed to die--sometimes slowly--or is not saved, and an active posture, where the baby would be killed. These distinctions are meaningless. Moreover, the dialog itself has a damaging effect because it hides the real issue.

Delayed personhood policy. There is a fifth option, which lies close to the second extreme we posed: Society could accept the benefits of extended technology, be unwilling to change the definition of human life or murder by legislation, and yet take cognizance of potential hardships and allow the relevant actors--principally the parents--considerable leeway to make individual decisions. Substantial sanctions thus would not be withheld. Under this model, the state could specifically reserve to parents of newborns who fall in a described category, the power to make balancing decisions about whether or not to continue the child's life. The state could do this without drastically altering the model definitions of life, although it might be necessary to have both definitional safeguards and policies about briefly withholding birth certificates and names from high risk infants and those in certain categories. In this way, diagnosis and evaluation could be more complete and parents better informed. Further, we might have an open, but saving, fiction of non-personhood,[20] and we could make abstracted decisions.

This model is, in many ways, like present abortion policy. The state does not now say that it is good to have abortions, only that it is permissible if the

mother judges that is what she wants. Nor does the
abortion policy necessarily change the ethic of having
babies. Allowing abortion does not cancel maternal
urges. There are natural limiters to the permissive
policy the state can rely on. In the neonatology decision, the universe of relevant parents includes only
those who have elected to carry a baby to term. Particularly with permissive abortion, the scales are
weighted heavily in favor of sustaining the baby who is
born.

We will urge serious consideration of the non-
personhood policy, because it is consistent with the
rest of the law of childhood where the state is forced
to trust parents to make the right decisions simply because they are in the best position to do so and because they have the most interest in outcomes and can
be given the pertinent information. Parents are now
able to make decisions about whether a baby will be
(*Roe v. Wade*) and what a child will be. Parents are
seen as relevant decisionmakers, and this delegation
subsumes a degree of risk that they will make both
"right" decisions and "wrong" decisions. The proposed
model can be located within this context.

A model for discussion. Paradoxically, what we
propose as a model for discussion lies close to the
Dunlap model (case-by-case decision, noted above),
which we reject. The difference lies in encouragement
or discouragement of individual decisionmaking. It
lies in making a policy decision, like many we already
make, that someone at the point of the agonizing dilemma--
be it the parents, the doctors, or someone else like the
judges--will know what is best to do under the individual circumstances. Our policy model would encourage
a common law development rather than simply allowing
decisionmaking to happen and at the same time dis-
couraging it from happening. We will return to the
balance of this discussion after we have identified
interests, actors, and capacities.

One final macro-observation. Again abortion is
seen as a crucial key to understanding the issues.
For some parents or would-be parents the decision to
abort may be based on amniocentesis and genetic counselling. What of parents who did not receive such assistance? Should this represent their last clear
chance? Or is it possible to view euthanasia in some
instances as a late abortion decision in much the same
way that abortion has been viewed as a late birth control decision?

Micro-Decision Alternatives

The decisions made in each individual case will
depend, of course, to a large degree on prevailing
public policy, i.e. on the previous macro-decisions.
Presently, with a restrictive policy, decisions are
made in individual hardship cases; they avoid the
dilemma imposed by fixed prohibitive policy and the
reality of substandard life. As we have noted, decisions are now made to depart from a standard of
life-saving at any cost. The departures are covert
and the actors are often battered by conflicts between
their acts and the announced prevailing ethic.

The decisions made covertly today under mercy
fictions may cost more than we now know. Each individual actor's burden of guilt, complicity and second-
guessing may be multiplied many times over. More important, there is a persistent tug-of-war as to who
are the relevant actors, who bears responsibility and
who sees reality. The result is unevenness. Decisions
depend on the moment, on opportunity and lack of opportunity, and to a large degree on actors arrogating
to themselves authority that is not or may not be
theirs.

Decisions out of time-phase. The policy of no
policy has another important consequence related to
timing. Assuming that there is presently good communication between doctors and patients about probabilities

of permanent defect (to the extent that doctors are able to make these estimates), the time for optimal "non-action" under today's ethic and the time for reflective communication are out of phase.

At the time of birth, and at the time that operating consents are needed, the medical team members are required by their ethic and by the habit of their training to move ahead without debate. Yet, paradoxically, this is the time that society most tolerates "losing" a child. Later, when there is time for evaluation, opportunity for such loss has passed. Our best technicians are ill-equipped to be our judges when the maximums of their techniques are required. Later, when the technicians can be of invaluable assistance to those who must make the decisions, their judgments are not tolerable or tolerated.

Policy or fiction. No matter what overall policy is adopted by society, the real decisions will still be made on a case-by-case basis. The nature of the predictions about a specific infant will always, and should always, remain crucial. Equally crucial is the understanding by the decisionmaker of the factors being balanced. There will always be a dilemma. The difference between affirmative policy and fiction, however, has to do with allocation of responsibility for making the decisions, assurances that the relevant interests are being balanced, and assurances that those who have the direct interests and will bear the costs are involved in the decisionmaking process.

QUESTION III:

Whose interests are involved?

Overall social decisions and specific on-the-spot decisions will, to a great extent, be a function of a cost-benefit analysis. The broader policy will comprise a relatively complex balancing of interests, while specific decisionmaking will be more directly related to the cost-benefit perceptions of those who are involved with the actual decision; it will be a function of the decisionmaker's estimate of his or her interests and his or her perception of the interests of others. Consider *Roe v. Wade* again. The court decision is a balancing of social, familial, and child interests, while the result of the decision requires that a pregnant female consider her interests, her family's interests, and the fetal interest *from her perspective*. To understand what may or may not be balanced, let us see if we can identify interests and actors.

The Baby

This is at once the most relevant actor and the most relevant interest and at the same time the most remote. When, in the next section we consider decisionmaking capacity, it is clear that the baby has none. But the baby's remoteness does not end with voice. The baby may be seen as a being distinct from its parents, but is not seen at all as having interests distinct from those articulated by its parents or by the state.[21]

Children occupy a status relationship. Accordingly, we have a resultant view of their wish to live with defects, or their wish to die. The dialog about operating consents and blood transfusions has always been one where, although the child was separately represented, the parents and the state competed as to who would speak to the child's interests.[22] *Roe v. Wade*, too, had this configuration for fetal interest.

Defining the child's best interests. Of some passing interest to us here are two kidney transplant cases involving children (not infants). In *Hart v. Brown*, 289 A. 2d 386 (Conn. Superior Court, 1972), the court considered whether a parent could consent to the donation of a kidney from a healthy seven-year-old to her failing identical twin. The court allowed the consent.[23] But the point here is that the overall interest

of the child was viewed as being articulated by a combination of the parents and the courts; the donor's
wishes were only projected images. In *Howard v. Fulton-
DeKalb Hospital Authority* (Superior Court of Fulton
County, Georgia, No. B-90430, November 29, 1973) the
court allowed a consent for a kidney transplant from
a 15-year-old mentally retarded girl to her mother.
The court reasoned that it would have to give consent,
because the mother had a competing interest (her own
health). The basis of the court's ruling, however,
was that the girl's interest was best served by the
survival of her mother. Again, the main point here
is the projection of interests. We may talk about the
child's interests as distinct, but they are resultant
from our definitions of the child's "best interests."

The child's voice. Here, of course, we are looking at the extreme situation, but the frame of analysis
remains the same. If we say that the child wants to
live or that the child wants to die, we have to recognize that we are listening to ourselves, to the immediate responses of the parents, the physicians, and others
directly involved, and to our cultural heritage and
biological persistence. What we will be hearing in the
voice of the child will be our own anguished mix of
frustration, commitment, and sentimentality. The child
has an interest, but it is what parents, community and
state, and doctors say it is.

The State

The state, too, has a direct interest--an interest
in the preservation of our collective symbols. But,
like the child, the interests of the state are projected
abstractions. The voice of the state, like the voice
of the child, is resultant. Collective will and collective myths are involved.

Order and costs. The state has two kinds of interests. First, it has an interest in the maintenance of
order and continuity; part of this interest relates to

preserving the nuclear family. Second, the state has
an interest in the economic and social costs of maintaining life--in or out of institutions--where those
who are initially charged with the burdens are unable
or unwilling to carry them. The state, in other words,
as a collective is the ultimate beneficiary or guaran-
tor of a given policy. It speaks to economic and
social benefits and costs.

The state's interest is not limitless. Indeed,
as we have seen in *Roe v. Wade*, the precise holding
of the court was that the state had no interest in the
first trimester of pregnancy, and little interest in
the second trimester. Part of this holding must be
attributed to the finding that there was no infant
voice to which the state could annex its concern--
personhood arose in the third trimester. The "right
to life" symbol that the state was trying to maintain
in anti-abortion statutes was held subordinate to the
interests of parents and siblings. The state also had
a countervailing interest in maintaining parental interest.

The state has an interest in maintaining a rule
against murder. But, again, these rules are not absolutes. Consider war, the death penalty, or numerous
policy discussions--such as highway safety--where life
is spent as part of known cost, i.e., a currency. We
know that we are dealing with extremely important values where a child has been born alive, albeit defective.
The interest of the state both in symbols and in direct
costs will not be dismissed as easily in the neonatology
euthanasia issues as they were in *Roe*. Much depends on
how important and persistent the particularized interests of the other actors are found to be. One way of
putting the state's concern gets us to the other half
of the state's dual interest: Does the state have an
interest in maintaining the lives of defective children?

The state and unwanted children. The state is not
new to the business of dealing with unwanted children.
Laws of child neglect, abuse, and dependency are based

on the assumption that where parents fail, the state takes over. The costs of present systems of foster care, hospitalization, and institutionalization of children are enormous whether reckoned in terms of state budgets or in child-centered terms that underscore the inadequacy of such arrangements. Educational costs are involved too.

What are the costs of additional defective children? In answering, we must not only assess economic costs, but also psychological costs to the society auditing its own solutions to its perceived problems, or society auditing the costs of non-solutions. What is the cost of a persistent nightmare?

If a policy were adopted that would change existing rules, the state would have an interest in accommodating as much change as was seen necessary to meet a problem, while at the same time maintaining as much continuity as possible.

The Parents

This is the first set of active, in personam, parties we have considered. (The other set of active participants is the medical staff.) The parents' interests are, for the most part, evident. The parents' hopes are involved. So, too, is the frustration of their hopes. They can view the child as a benefit or a burden. They can view themselves as enriched or enslaved, rewarded or punished. The parents have an interest in the existing family, including the interests of siblings.

The parents also have an important economic interest at stake. As the law now stands, the primary burden of maintaining and supporting the child belongs to them. Even where part of the burden is shifted to the state, the existing ethic involves the institutionalization of *their* child, the state supporting *their* child, with the state asking for support from parents. Psychological costs are annexed to these arrangements.

Ability to nurture. Economic costs, however, are the smaller part of the problem. The crucial interest involved is how the parents relate or will relate to the child. Implicit in the legal expectations about the parent-child relationship, and implicit in the social expectations undergirding the legal arrangements, is a view that parents will supply something beyond material comfort and protection. At some level the parents will be expected to nurture the child, and they will expect themselves to nurture the child. To the extent that they can do this, they have a wanted child; to the extent that they cannot, they have an unwanted child. We have already observed some of the similarities between the neonatology problem and the abortion problem. Most of the parental interests involved are identical.

The parents have an interest in speaking for the child. But as we have already observed, whether the child be normal or defective, it is difficult to say when if ever the parents see the child's interests as distinct from theirs.

The Medical Staff

As the other set of active participants in the neonatology dilemma, the medical staff has distinct interests, too--both professional and personal. The medical staff has an interest in good medicine, in the art of healing, in the avoidance of harm, and in the maintenance of symbols and standards that further these aims and enable the staff to like themselves as well. They want to practice good medicine and be committed to what they are doing.

Need for guidelines. The dilemma we are examining arises out of a quantum jump in technology that alters the definitions of life-saving, and of life itself. A fixed star, life-saving at all costs, has dropped out of the medical constellation. Of primary interest to the medical staff, therefore, is the search for new operating guidelines--new navigational aids. The guidelines must invite the utmost commitment (as did the Hippocratic Oath) and the good practice of medicine, and also inhibit recklessness and indifference.

The medical staff has somewhat the same problems as parents and the state: how to articulate, for others, their own interests. Is the medical profession articulating its interest, the interests of the patient, or the interests of the state? Does the medical staff seek to speak for the infant? This would be natural. But what are the consequences? Who is the patient? The infant or the parents? We are asking more probing questions here than simply who has the legal right to consent or withhold consent for treatment. For what interest is the medical team a surrogate?

Keeping interests separate. Professional and personal interests are often hard to keep separate, even when it is desirable to do so. For the loving pediatricians I have seen, I am glad this is true. It is important, however, to understand at what point one's personal predilection is mixing with professional interest. For a professional lacking this understanding, the results can be awesome. It must be remembered that the other active participants have a role, too, but that it is not professionalized. There are no professional parents.

Finally, the medical profession stands in a distinctly different place with respect to burdens. There are short-run burdens on the medical team--excruciating and haunting burdens. The long-run costs--economic and psychological--do not fall on the medical staff, however. They fall on the infant, the parents, and the state (society-at-large).

QUESTION IV:

Decision-making capacities and opportunities: who can decide and who should decide?

In this paper, we have repeatedly shunted aside an assumption we should now face. Are there babies in the intensive care units that can be reliably identified as unable to develop into normal human beings? If there are, how much certainty do we require? How much abnormality is unacceptable? What should be done about those situations where we are reasonably sure but hesitate to act? Who should make the decisions? More important, who should take the risks? Some of the answers to these questions, of course, relate to the ultimate overall policy decisions that society makes.

The point here is to face whether we are talking about *certainty* or *high risk*. Again, an analogy to the abortion field is in order. Even pre-*Roe v. Wade*, when therapeutic abortion was allowed, the decision to abort where the prospective mother had rubella in the first trimester was based not on certainty but on the high probability of deformity. Recognizing that we are now dealing with identified human babies, how much greater certainty are we asking for? Will there not always be some risk that the "wrong" decision is made?

Imperative Solutions or Permissible Solutions

We started here because we have to face whether we are talking about imperative solutions or permissible solutions. If we were talking about a narrow range of babies about whom we were certain, perhaps we could say that medical diagnosis and decisionmaking are one and the same; we could perhaps define a category of babies who should be *killed* independent of the wishes of any of the actors. But we are in fact discussing situations where the diagnoser and prognosticator can only make estimates of probability of subnormality, of the need for continued intensive care, or of the need for institutionalization if the baby lives. Under these circumstances if we allow someone to make the decision, we have to face early the fact that the decision is not a medical or scientific decision, but rather a social decision, a decision that calls for balancing. This, in part, involves issues of timing.

Timing

As things now stand, and as we have already pointed out, the optimal social time for "letting a baby go" is in the first few hours. But this is the time when the medical team knows the least and is least able to take the time to evaluate the situation. The commands of medical training and commitment are to proceed with haste to maintain viability, to refrain from judging. In the process, decisions are made because options have been closed out. The doctors have become the decision-makers, because they were the only ones with opportunity. Now vary the equation slightly, and say that society permits a reflective decision--that maintaining the viability in the first few hours or the first few days preserves rather than eliminates options. Can we say that the doctors are now the only ones who have the opportunity to make a decision or have the paramount interest in making the decision? That appears doubtful, because the medical facts are only one of the factors that have to be balanced, and the medical team either is unaware of all of the other--social--factors of the decision, or they have no direct interest in such factors.

Parents and Meaningful Decisions

Under present arrangements lack of meaningful parental opportunity is another factor that should be noted. Not only are parents excluded from decision-making by reason of the need for speed, already noted, but, if they are aware of defects and "high risk," we

may say that they are too traumatized to make a meaningful decision. The parents are therefore either
swept along by hope or memory of hope, or they feel
the pressure of the prevailing life-saving ethic.
Under these circumstances, parents are not decisionmakers; yet they are the biggest stake holders. They
are the ones taking the risks of burdens. In a significant sense, their lives are on the line.

Again, vary the equation slightly. Suppose that
reflective judgment is permitted. Would parents then
have a meaningful opportunity to make decisions? Or,
more exactly, could we then view the parents as capable
of making meaningful decisions? We have entered the
precincts of informed consent and choices about who are
the interested decisionmakers.

Under a policy of reflective judgment--permissive
policy to allow neonates to die of uncorrected anomalies or to allow the taking of their lives--would not
the relationship of the doctor and the patient change,
particularly if the parent is seen as the relevant
decisionmaker?[24] There would be an opportunity to
blend an understanding of the medical outlook with an
understanding of the other factors to be balanced.
The medical team would have an opportunity to explain
the "facts" and be supportive, allowing the parents to
make judgments with an informed heart. This, of course,
assumes that the other actors would view the parents
as the relevant decisionmakers.

Parents and balancing decisions. Let's back up.
Is there any question that the parents, under a reflective scheme, are the only ones who have sufficient interests to make the balancing decisions required? Are
the parents in a different position from the mother
in *Roe v. Wade*? Is the medical team in a different
position? Do the medical people have a direct interest in the outcome? The parents are the only ones in
a position to make the intimate trade-offs--costs,
family displacements, assessments of their own readiness for the burdens, and assessments about their own
lives vs. the life of the defective infant.

Articles of faith. In essence, the choice of parents as decisionmakers in other than emergency situations comes down to two articles of faith: (1) trust in the parents' abilities to understand the medical probabilities, and (2) trust in the parents to make a better judgment than anyone else. The first point is relatively easy: as in all informed consent, what the parents know is a function of what the doctor tells them. When there is insufficient time to communicate, or where the physician is guarded in what he tells the parents--for reasons of professional self-image or personal predilections about what is the "right" thing to do--the resulting consent is not informed consent. What informed consent may come down to in the neonatology dilemma is shared reality--an assessment of what is known and what is not known--and shared horror.

The second article of faith is more complex. It involves a trust of ourselves. At the end of this long paper, we will simply remind the reader of the assumptions and factors of this trust. It is a reiteration: Society now trusts parents in many total ways. Parents decide whether a child will be, and what they hope a child will be. The present neonatology dilemma in fact, appears to be a window between (a) absolute autonomy over the decision of whether to carry to term and (b) an extensive range of personality molding and even physique molding decisions--such as balanced nutrition or unbalanced nutrition--that the parents are permitted to make.

The present policy--the window--seems in part to reflect a mystique surrounding birth. It is a legitimate mystique but a mystique nonetheless: we are present at the creation. But, now, with *Roe v. Wade* behind us, and with the "right to die" dialog well on the way, perhaps we are ready to demystify our reality. Society not only invented its children, it has invented the rest of its reality, too. Perhaps we are ready to face our own processes and to trust them.[25]

CONCLUSION

As this paper was started, we envisioned a final section on safeguards against recklessness. We envisioned an audit process by the courts, recognizing that parents' interests could be seen to conflict with the interests of society and the child. We now have some problems. We have difficulty seeing that the courts, in a prospective sense, can bring a better wisdom to bear than that of parents. Further, we see the possibility of the mythology of "right" decisions persisting if courts were involved in a pre-audit of decisionmaking. Abstract decisions would be substituted for personal, specific decisions. We fear the personal predilections of judges almost as much as we fear the predilections of doctors. Part of this reaction is tutored by our observations of other instances of judicial intervention into the family decisionmaking process, notably the juvenile court.[26] The benign, reflective intent of actors who have only "the best interests of the children" in mind frequently turn into nightmares, more frequently than not. Faced with the dilemma that faces parents of defective children, who can be their judges?

It is unrealistic to assume, however, that the present policy will change without safeguards. Since this is the case, we would prefer a system of post-audit. We would prefer a system that broadly defined the class of infants who could be disposed of by their parents, a system that did not require certainty, that could then be coupled with criminal sanctions for actions taken against children who fall outside the category.

This suggestion is more loving than at first may be apparent. Societal health and survival rely heavily on the reproductive urges and instincts. It also relies heavily on the willingness of parents to nurture their young. When this willingness disappears, it cannot be coerced from outside--it cannot be coerced by the state.

Paradoxically, allowing parents to accept the responsibility and the consequences of their own choices with respect to their children may produce a greater number of mature, willing parents, not a lesser number. We believe that the abortion decision--*Roe v. Wade*--is based on an innate understanding of this paradox.

Views on the Ethics of Infant Euthanasia

Michael J. Garland[*]

INTRODUCTION

Professional ethicists have begun to take up the
questions raised by the life-sustaining capabilities of
neonatal medicine. They are seeking to identify the
reasons offered as justification for initiating, continuing or withholding therapeutic efforts on a defective newborn. Some philosophers and theologians attempt
to identify guidelines for deciding in individual cases
whether one ought or ought not to continue therapy.
Others examine elements in the wider social context
that might justifiably pre-set such decisions.

This paper reviews articles by six ethicists who
have explicitly addressed the question of *infant* euthanasia rather than the broader topic of euthanasia in
general. These writings were chosen also because they
explore several philosophic concepts that are presumably
applicable to the problem: the right to life, the unjust aggressor, due process, authority, personhood,
obligation, fairness, values, and the use of ordinary
and extraordinary means for prolonging life. Surveying
the articles together may help the reader assess the

[*]Lecturer in Bioethics, School of Medicine, University
of California, San Francisco.

usefulness of these tools of ethical analysis in dealing with the problems raised in this volume. No attempt has been made either to argue with these authors or to pit their positions against each other.

TOOLEY: INFANTICIDE AND THE RIGHT TO LIFE

In his article "Abortion and Infanticide,"[1] philosopher Michael Tooley argues that infanticide is a generally justifiable act. The argument rests on his demonstration that newborn infants do not have a right to life and may therefore be allowed to die during a relatively short period soon after birth (a week is suggested as a reasonable, though admittedly arbitrary, cutoff point). He links the rationales for infanticide and abortion in response to a common criticism of the liberal position on abortion. He notes, "Reasons adduced in justification of abortion also justify infanticide; but since people generally reject infanticide as evil, so also should abortion be rejected." Tooley accepts the moral uniformity of the two actions but attempts to show that a forthright argument justifying infanticide is possible and, indeed, provides the only adequate basis for arguments in favor of abortion. In addition, Tooley indicates that this approach to abortion also settles the practical problem of whether or not one is obliged to keep defective newborns alive.

Asking what constitutes the "right to life", Tooley answers that an organism has a serious right to life only if it possesses the concept of the self as a continuing subject of experiences and other mental states and believes itself to be such a continuing entity. Infanticide is justified, he says, because newly born infants cannot meet these criteria and therefore need not be considered possessors of a serious right to life.

The Meaning of a Right

The argument begins with an initial consideration of what it means to have rights. Rights are essentially conditional. They depend on the existence of certain desires in the individual to whom the right is ascribed. To have a right to something therefore means that others have a prima facie obligation not to deprive the subject of his rightful possession as long as he desires it.

In humans, says Tooley, the right to life does not mean merely continued biological existence, but continued existence as a subject of experiences and other mental states. Therefore, the expression "right to life" with respect to humans presupposes that the individual is a subject capable of experiences and other mental states. And since rights are conditioned by desires, right to life presupposes that the individual desires to continue to live as a subject of experience (a self). But a desire is the wish that certain propositions be true, e.g., "I wish it to be true that I will continue to exist." To have this wish is to be capable of forming the concepts that constitute the proposition. The key concept in this proposition is the concept of the self as a continuing subject of experiences, an "I". An entity that lacks this self-consciousness cannot have a right to life.

Thus, Tooley arrives at his dual requirement for a serious right to life: (1) self-consciousness and (2) the desire to continue existing as a self.

The Desire to Continue

He observes that emotional disturbance might temporarily destroy the desire to continue existing as a self. The desire would also appear to be absent during temporary unconsciousness. And it is conceivable that one might be maliciously *conditioned* to no longer desire to exist as a self. These exceptions, according to Tooley, indicate that the right is conditioned not only by actual

desire but by presumptive or constructed desires. It
is reasonable to presume that an individual *would* desire
to continue living as a self were he not disturbed emotionally, or temporarily unconscious, or conditioned to
no longer desire existing as a self. However, none of
these exceptions fits the case of the infant whose capacity for concepts and desire for continued existence are
not temporarily interrupted or externally manipulated
but simply not yet actual.

With his theoretical argument thus completed, Tooley
faces the factual questions: When do members of the
species homo sapiens acquire the self-consciousness requisite for possessing a serious right to life? It is
not clear when this happens, but it clearly does not
happen until some time after birth and arguably before
the acquisition of language. Although it is troublesome
theoretically to determine where the line is to be drawn,
it is not a practical problem since most desirable in-
fanticides can take place shortly after birth, probably
within the first week.

Tooley's argument resolves the dilemma of letting
defective newborns die. They have no right to life, he
says, and parents may justifiably rid themselves of the
burden they represent.

SMITH: FOR THE INFANT'S SAKE...OR FOR SOMEONE ELSE'S?

David H. Smith, a theologian, discusses two kinds
of questions in his article "On Letting Some Babies
Die."[2] First are the procedural questions about who
has the authority to decide whether or not to terminate
a life. The second set concerns the grounds for the
decision, whether it is primarily for the sake of the
infant or for the sake of others.

Smith sets his discussion in the context of a prima
facie prohibition of killing human persons and the pre-
sumption that the infants in question *are* human persons

to whom this prohibition applies. He notes that not every product of the human womb is such a person. The prohibition would not apply, perhaps, to a child born without a developed brain (anencephalic).

The family or parents are the appropriate locus of the primary authority to make such a decision. They should be supported and counselled in this by physicians. However, since the infant cannot decide for himself, those who decide must do so under the rule of acting in the infant's best interests which, he cautions, need not be simply equated with prolonged life.

The Interest of Others

The commonly urged grounds for the decision to let a baby die are examined in two categories: those that appeal to the interests of the infant and those that appeal to the interests of others. When the interests of others are appealed to, Smith suggests, some analogy of a "just war theory" is at work. The infant is seen as an aggressor threatening harm to some other person or group. But if this line of argument is to be used, he charges, it must be complete.

It must be shown that the infant brings actual threat against specified persons, that the solution of the infant's death is a solution of last resort (all other possible means of evading his presumed threat having been attempted or examined and found ineffectual). It must be shown also that some form of due process has been provided the infant (some uninvolved party having verified that there is a real threat and that the infant's death is indeed a solution of last resort). These criteria, Smith argues, can rarely, if ever, be fulfilled in an affluent society, particularly the criterion of last resort.

The Infant's Interest

The second common justification for infant euthanasia is that of the infant's own interests. Here death is considered better for the infant than continued life because of the quality of life to be lived (e.g., handicapped, disfigured, retarded). Smith would allow certain rare, perhaps hypothetical, instances where these grounds might justify euthanasia (probably active as well as passive euthanasia). Thus he would consider it appropriate to cease trying to cure an infant in whom the dying process had irretrievably begun. He also cites permanent unconsciousness and intractable pain as conditions justifying infant euthanasia (perhaps even active euthanasia).

Smith criticizes many contemporary arguments for infant euthanasia because they slide back and forth between these two justifying grounds without achieving adequacy on either basis. He concludes that the infant euthanasia decision is rarely justifiable on the grounds of the child's best interests, and practically never justifiable on the grounds of someone else's interests (at least in an affluent society).

However, as an addendum Smith indicates that the proportion of defective persons in society need not be increased by adherence to his position. That proportion can be controlled by public policy decisions of resource allocation. By limiting the resources allocated for the provision of "heroic" neonatal care the number of defective survivors is not likely to grow. Selection for such care should be done on the basis of either random choice or "first-come, first-served." This argument, Smith notes, presumes that salvaging defective newborns may not be our highest priority. It is offered as an alternative to choosing among endangered newborns at the individual level on any basis other than first-come, first-served.

GUSTAFSON: PARENTAL DESIRES AND
THE RIGHT TO LIFE

Theologian James M. Gustafson in "Mongolism, Parental Desires, and the Right to Life"[3] discusses the case of a mongoloid infant with an operable intestinal blockage (duodenal atresia), who was allowed to die because his parents chose not to permit corrective surgery.

His method was to analyze the context of the event, examine the values and moral principles present in the decisions of the relevant participants and compare these with his own concepts. He found that his own views would lead to the decision to operate and save the child's life.

The general context may be summarized as one in which the parents and doctors had to decide about a relatively safe surgical procedure that would save the infant's life without changing the fact of mongoloid handicap. The parents were white, middle class, a lawyer and a nurse, and had two previous normal children. This decision took place in a cultural setting where there were legal means to seek to override the parental decision in order to perform the life-saving procedure.

Gustafson found the maternal decision to be basically guided by negative feelings about having a mongoloid. These feelings supported the desire to let the child die rather than take surgical means to keep it alive. In part these feelings and the desire were informed by her sense of fairness--it wouldn't be fair to the other children to raise the mongoloid child together with them.

The father seemed merely to go along with the position taken by the mother.

Evaluating Mongolism

The physicians' compliance with the parental decision was influenced by their perception of mongolism as

an abnormal, defective condition. If the child were
normal and needing the same operation they would have
sought a court order in response to parental refusal to
allow the operation. They expressed the opinion that
the court would not have ordered the operation on a mongoloid child. However, they took the position that active euthanasia would be wrong.

Gustafson noted that the nurses expressed frustration with the decision but had to follow it. Moreover,
they were powerless to alter it since they could not
perform the required surgery.

In analyzing the situation, Gustafson noted that
the key was the value placed on normal intelligence by
the parents, the physicians, and presumptively, the
courts. Since the mongoloid could certainly not have
normal intelligence it was judged permissible to let
him die. Crucially, this valuation seems to account
for the non-attribution to the mongoloid child of a
right to life.

Gustafson's method does not yield a precise guideline for deciding if and when some infants might be allowed to die, but provides indicators that may be applicable to other settings.

Summary of Indicators

First, says Gustafson, the fact that an infant is
alive and dependent is of crucial importance. The dependency of infants accounts for the fact that all parents have the *power* to decide whether the infant shall
continue to live. This power does not confer the *right*
to decide whether the infant shall live or die on the
basis of one's negative feelings and desires about him.
Rather, as a general rule, the existence and dependence
of an infant obligate parents and others to provide support and nurture. Obligations of parents and physicians
toward any child are grounded in his existence and

dependent state, not in the desires of others to keep and rear him. (Gustafson would except genetic monstrosities from the field of obligation for vital support).

Second, mongoloids have a number of qualities and potentialities that make their lives valuable both to themselves and to others. Although they have subnormal intelligence they are capable of personal happiness and a wide range of human relationships including the capacity to give and receive love. These potentialities outweigh the handicap of subnormal intelligence.

Third, the suffering that a mongoloid would presumably cause parents and siblings is judged by Gustafson to be tolerable. Thousands of other families are able to bear it. Thus it does not seem so great that one might justifiably avoid it at the cost of another's life.

Fourth, Gustafson points to the altruistic ethic urged in the Judaeo-Christian tradition. This theme gives a bias toward dealing with problem-persons, such as defective newborns, by accepting considerable inconvenience and cost to oneself in seeking the well-being of "the other."

McCORMICK: SURVIVAL AND THE POTENTIAL FOR HUMAN RELATIONSHIPS

Jesuit theologian Richard A. McCormick, in "To Save or Let Die"[4] observes an emerging fact of neonatal medicine: There are some infants many agree ought to be saved in spite of illness or deformity, while there are others many agree ought to be allowed to die. This fact, he judges, implies that an explicit guideline for making such decisions can and ought to be identified.

McCormick believes a guideline may be developed by examining the basis for the widely used distinction between ordinary means of preserving life and health (taken to be obligatory) and extraordinary means (taken to be nonobligatory). Implicit in this distinction is the

concept that life is a basic good to be preserved not
for its own sake but as a condition for realizing other
values or higher spiritual goods. These latter values
establish both the duty to preserve physical life and
the limits of such duty. Thus, life is to be preserved
if realization of the higher goods will still be possible
for the survivor.

To give substance to the guideline, McCormick draws
on the view of man that is basic to the Judaeo-Christian
tradition: The higher spiritual goods are love of God
and love of neighbor, with love of God expressed in love
of neighbor. Thus the meaning, substance, and consum-
mation of life are found in human relationships sur-
rounded by qualities of justice, respect, concern, com-
passion and support. The guideline thus would state
that life is to be preserved if human relationships will
still be possible for the survivor.

Positively, the guideline provides the test: If
it survives will this infant retain some potential for
human relationships? Several negative test formulations
are used: Will the potential for human relationships be
totally absent or totally subordinated to the mere effort for survival? Will it be "totally submerged and
undeveloped in the mere struggle for survival" and "de-
void of any meaningful relational potential"? In the
case of a negative status, the infant may be said to
have "achieved its potential" and therefore may be allowed to die.

McCormick posts six caveats around this guideline:

1. To guide "gray area" decisions, physicians must
try to identify those biologic conditions that probably
provide negative indicators (e.g., a baby born without
a brain has no relational potential, while a mongoloid
has such potential.)

2. It is better to err on the side of sustaining
life.

3. All lives are to be valued, even those whose absent or submerged potential for relationship calls for allowing death.

4. Parents and physicians should not decide on the basis of the child's usefulness or productive capacity.

5. Decisions must be made in terms of the child's good alone.

6. The Judaeo-Christian imperative to cherish and protect the weak urges preservation of infant lives as long as infants can experience caring and love.

FLETCHER: THE SOCIAL CONSEQUENCES OF INFANT EUTHANASIA

In "Abortion, Euthanasia, and Care of Defective Newborns"[5] theologian John Fletcher inquires if judgments about the morality of aborting defective fetuses are useful guides in questions of euthanasia of defective newborns. (He uses "euthanasia" strictly in the sense of mercy killing.) He notes that some ethicists on opposite sides of the abortion debate agree that the moral norms for abortion and infant euthanasia are the same.

He cites the positions of two such ethicists, Paul Ramsey[6] and Joseph Fletcher.[7] Ramsey holds that arguments for abortion equally justify infanticide. If, therefore, we would not accept infanticide, we should not do abortions (except in rare instances where the mother's life is at stake). Joseph Fletcher argues in the opposite direction: Abortion of defective fetuses is an accepted good; therefore, the morally identical act of euthanasia of defective newborns is likewise good.

Application of Norms

John Fletcher argues that the prenatal and postnatal situations are not morally identical. What is normative for one situation should not be considered normative for the other. While it is good to abort defective fetuses, it is wrong to practice euthanasia on defective newborns. Three empirical differences between the situations support his position. First, the separate physical existence of the infant after birth confronts parents, physicians and others with independent moral claims for care and support. Second, after birth, disease in the infant is available to physicians for therapy. Third, parental acceptance of the infant is more developed at birth than at earlier stages of pregnancy. These three differences, Fletcher urges, signify that even if defective, the newborn is a fellow human being, deserving protection on legal and ethical grounds.

Fletcher adds two further reasons for opposing infant euthanasia: It is potentially brutalizing for the "killer;" and if society were to accept and legalize the killing of defective newborns, it would undermine the optimal conditions for beginning life--the child's experience of trust in his parents and the world.

Passive Euthanasia

While Fletcher is opposed to mercy killing, he notes that there are cases of terribly damaged newborns for whom death is the desirable outcome. Therapy for the defect may not be available or would only prolong the agony of the dying process. In such cases the infant should be allowed to die by withholding support while relieving pain. He judges that the self-restraint of passive euthanasia is consistent with the legal and ethical norm,binding both parents and physicians: "Do no harm."

Fletcher sees and recognizes empirical differences between the fetus and the newborn and recognizes the cultural values (religious and secularist) of the inherent dignity of each member of the human family. These recognitions provide his basis for prohibition of infant euthanasia and distinguish the issue from the morality of aborting defective fetuses.

ENGELHARDT: THE DUTY NOT
TO PROLONG LIFE

Physician-philosopher, H. Tristram Engelhardt, Jr.
proposes a new ethical concept, "the injury of continued
existence" in "Ethical Issues in Aiding the Death of
Young Children."[8] He combines this concept with the
medical ethics dictum, "Do no harm," to establish a duty
not to sustain life in cases where only a short, painful, or marginal existence could follow.

This position argues that it is in the individual's
interest not to live a short, painful, compromised life.
To force such a life on an infant is to do harm to him;
thus the duty is not to prolong life in such cases.
Engelhardt has in mind passive euthanasia (not resisting
death). Active euthanasia (direct killing), although
justified in particular cases, would be socially impru-
dent as a general rule because it is likely to erode the
status of children in general.

Rights, Obligations, Consequences

Not all cases of justifiable infant euthanasia can
be handled by this rule. It applies only in the cases
of inevitably brief, painful or intellectually marginal
life. Engelhardt indicates Tay-Sachs and Lesch-Nyhan
babies as typical cases where the duty not to prolong
life would certainly apply.[*] The more extensive category of defective newborn who might justifiably be allowed to die must be approached on other grounds.

Engelhardt indicates that the euthanasia of infants
(and young children) involves questions of the rights

----

[*]
 Tay-Sachs disease is inherited and usually leads to
death by age three or four. The lives of such infants
manifest increasing spasticity and dementia. Lesch-
Nyhan disease is marked by mental retardation and com-
pulsive self-mutilation.

of children, the rights of parents, societal obligations toward the young and the societal consequences of euthanasia of young children.

The main problem is that young children are not yet persons in the strict sense, he says. They are not responsible moral agents who can be said to be bearers of rights and duties. Their existence is morally defined by and through familial interaction. To respect an infant is to hold in trust its existence so that it can develop as a moral person and later assume responsibility as a bearer of rights and duties.

Roles of Parents and Physicians

If this is the case, then the use of medical intervention to prolong the life of a critically ill infant should be evaluated from two aspects: in relation to the probability of future personal life for the infant, and in relation to the accompanying psychic and monetary costs to the parents. It is a decision within the ambit of parental authority. The physician's role is to provide sufficient information for the parents to make a reasoned choice. Engelhardt argues that there is no positive duty to treat the infant if the procedure is very costly or there is slim hope of success. These elements are usually combined in specific cases, but either is sufficient to justify a decision to let an infant die.

Society should intervene in such a parental decision only if the costs, psychic and monetary, would not constitute a severe burden on the parents and there is a strong likelihood of good quality of future life for the child. Engelhardt offers two rules for societal intervention into this sphere of parental authority: (1) when a decision to let an infant die is unreasonable and would undermine care for children generally; (2) when, in a parental decision to prolong a defective infant's life, intervention would prevent the child from suffering unnecessary pain.

CONCLUSION

The reader is invited to reflect on and evaluate the arguments presented here. A variety of approaches and methods of ethical inquiry are presented. By way of summary, they converge and differ in their response to the questions: "Would death be a justifiable choice to solve the problems associated with the birth of a defective infant? If so, on what grounds?" All of the authors agree that the infant's death is a morally justifiable choice for parents, physicians, or others to make--given the proper circumstances. But they vary significantly on the grounds for justification and the definition of the proper circumstances.

Tooley: Death is a justifiable solution because newborn children quite simply have no serious right to life.

Smith: Death is a justifiable solution (a) if the infant is truly an unjust aggressor giving actual threat to specified persons and his death is a solution of last resort determined by some form of due process; or (b) if death is truly in the best interests of the infant (e.g., the infant is irretrievably dying, or in intractable pain, or permanently unconscious). The number of surviving defective children can (should) be controlled by limiting the resources allocated for the work of salvaging endangered newborns.

Gustafson: Death is a justifiable solution if the full range of human potential in the infant is virtually zero and the burden imposed on others by the task of caring for it is judged intolerable.

McCormick: Death is a justifiable solution if the potential for human relationships is totally absent or totally subordinated to the mere effort for survival.

Fletcher: Death is a justifiable solution in the case of a seriously damaged newborn for whom death is the desirable outcome and the death is not accomplished by euthanasia. Euthanasia would brutalize the "killer" and undermine the social conditions necessary to enable newborns to develop basic trust in their parents and their world.

Engelhardt: Death is a justifiable (optional) solution if a defective child has a low probability for a future life of quality, or if the psychic and monetary costs to parents would constitute a severe burden. (Parents *may* decide against life-prolonging treatment.) Death is a justifiable (obligatory) solution if the child's life could be only briefly prolonged, or would be painful or marginal. (Parents *should* decide against life prolonging treatment.)

A Moral Policy for Life/Death Decisions in the Intensive Care Nursery

Albert R. Jonsen

and

Michael J. Garland*

INTRODUCTION

When individuals face decisions on matters about which they have moral convictions, they act in accord with those convictions, or they violate them, or find compromises, excuses or extenuating circumstances to resolve dilemmas. However, when many individuals with diverse moral convictions face a series of decisions about similar cases, there should be a way to accommodate the diversity of private beliefs with some degree of broad agreement about how such cases should be managed.

We call this effort making a moral policy.[1] Such a policy should describe not only substantive ethical principles to which the majority might agree, but also the social arrangements that would facilitate discussion

---

*
See also the writers' individual papers in this volume.

and action on the basis of those principles. Thus, a moral policy combines statements of both principle and procedure. The moral policy presents the elements of a reasonable ethical argument: certain rules; attributions of responsibility and duty; and medical, psychological, social and economic facts.

A word of warning: such a moral policy may seem unreal. This aspect is the inevitable result of considering moral decisions apart from the actualities of fear, self-interest and exhaustion, as well as from the dominance of some persons and the truancy of others charged with responsibility and duty. But the air of unreality provides, we believe, the necessary cool moment which philosophers say should precede any reasonable judgment. That judgment will have to be made amid hard realities, but it may be more clearly understood in the light of reflection on the following propositions.

ETHICAL PROPOSITIONS

1. Every baby born possesses a *moral value* that entitles it to the medical and social care necessary to effect its well-being.

2. Parents bear the principal *moral responsibility* for the well-being of their newborn infant.

3. Physicians have the *duty* to take medical measures conducive to the well-being of the baby in proportion to the relationships of trust or confidence they have with the parents.

4. The state has an *interest* in the proper fulfillment of responsibilities and duties regarding the well-being of the infant, as well as an interest in ensuring an equitable apportionment of limited resources among its citizens.

5.   The responsibility of the parents, the duty of the physician, and the interests of the state are conditioned by the medico-moral principle, "Do no harm, without expecting compensating benefit for the patient."

6.   Life-preserving intervention should be understood as doing harm to an infant who cannot survive infancy, or who will live in intractable pain, or who cannot participate even minimally in human experience.

7.   When courts are called upon to resolve disagreement among parents and physicians about medical care, prognosis about quality of life for the infant should weigh heavily in the decision as to whether or not to order life-saving intervention.

8.   In the final care of infants from whom life-sustaining support or curative efforts are withheld, analgesics should be used whenever indicated for avoiding pain, even though their use might hasten death.

9.   In cases of limited availability of neonatal intensive care, it is ethical to terminate therapy for an infant with poor prognosis in order to provide care for an infant with a much better prognosis.

COMMENTARY ON ETHICAL PROPOSITIONS

These propositions identify four moral "fields of force" that must be taken into account in decisions about sustaining neonatal life. Each field is designated by a term with strong ethical connotations: *moral value, responsibility, duty,* and *interest.* These terms suggest that the various parties in the neonatal situation have diverse roles and relationships. The metaphor "fields of force" implies that the parties each initiate, attract, or repel certain actions by reason of their moral relationships to one another.

Moral Fields of Force: The First Four Propositions

Moral value indicates that any living infant, even though unable to comprehend, decide, communicate, or defend his existence, must be approached with attitudes of respect, consideration, and care. The infant is designated a being in his own right endowed with moral autonomy. Although dependent on others for his survival, the infant's fundamental worth is not a function of how much or little others value him. He is independently valuable. This conception of the independent and equal value of human beings is basic in modern Western civilization. We assume its validity for our discussion and judge that the burden of proof lies on those who would deny it.

Responsibility signifies that those who engender and willingly bring an infant to birth are morally accountable for its well-being. They are closest to the infant, and must bear the burdens of its nurture, especially if it is ill or defective. This principle is stated with full recognition that some parents will not or cannot exercise this responsibility. Nonetheless, it states an ideal of the family in Western civilization and a demand that medical professionals should acknowledge in their attitudes and institutional arrangements.

Duty applies to the professional relationship of the physician[2] in attendance, who has two clients, the infant and the parents. The relationship is fiduciary, entered into freely by the physician with the parents who entrust their infant to the medical judgment of the physician for the sake of effecting the infant's well-being. Informed consent of the patient usually controls fiduciary relationships. Because the infant, who is the actual patient in this relationship, is unable to be a consenting partner, parental decisions normally control the relationship. But the physician, responding directly to the moral value of his infant-patient, may at times be duty-bound to resist a parental decision.

Physicians may feel that their duty extends not only to a particular infant under care but also to all children. Consequently, some physicians may be devoted to scientific research aimed at improving the quality and effectiveness of neonatal care for all. While this dedication is necessary and praiseworthy, it may at times influence decisions about the care of a particular patient. In the interest of scientific observation and data acquisition a clinician may, even unconsciously, be moved to extend care beyond reasonable limits set by the interest of the patient.

Interest designates the concern of society at large that individuals respect certain values and fulfill certain responsibilities and duties. Society also has an interest in the fair and efficient distribution of benefits as well as the promotion of health and well-being of its citizens. If promotion of the child's well-being unavoidably jeopardizes other equally worthy endeavors, a reconciliation of the competing interests must be sought. These concerns remain in the background unless a perceived threat to the common good requires remedial or preventive intervention.

"Fields of force" as a designation of parental responsibility, physician's duty and societal concern means that, morally, the ultimate decisions lie with the parents. This does not, however, mean that parents will always make those decisions. They may be absent physically or psychologically. They may even abdicate their moral right to make decisions by failure to be concerned with the well-being of the infant. In such cases, the physician's duty is expanded to include the heavy burden of final decisions.

We view the moral fields of force as attracting and repelling certain kinds of actions. Thus, the value of the infant attracts respect, consideration, and care; it repels indifference, violence, and neglect. Reponsibility attracts specific forms of care for the infant; it repels unconcern. The fields of force converge in decisions about neonatal survival, so that the valued infant is the focus of parental responsibility, physician duty, and state interest.[3] Each of these values has its limits; each is subordinate to the moral value of the infant. Responsibilities, duties, and interests require many specific actions. For example, it is the responsibility of parents to nourish the infant, the duty of the physician to cure the infant's illness, the interest of the state to punish neglect of the infant.

Do No Harm: The Fifth Proposition

We propose that the traditional medico-moral principle "Do no harm" is most appropriate to guide decisions regarding neonatal survival. Its appropriateness rests on the following considerations:

First, the principle, stated in the negative, admits of no exceptions. Positive formulations of moral obligation, such as "Preserve life," admit exceptions and must be qualified by listing grounds for them. The traditional medical principle, "Do no harm," is universally applicable. The problem, then, is not in finding grounds for exception but in defining harm.[4]

Second, while many medical interventions effect some harm, either transient or permanent, that harm is usually justified by an expected compensatory benefit. If no benefit can be reasonably expected, or if the benefit does not compensate for the harm, the intervention is unethical. Judgment about the likelihood of benefit rests with the physician; assessment of whether the benefit does compensate for the harm lies principally with the patient. In the case of infants, the assessment must be made by those who bear responsibility and duty within a context of broad medical and social understanding.

Intensive Care and Harm: The Sixth Proposition

Intensive care may in the context of certain life conditions, appear harmful. These conditions are identified as inability to survive infancy, inability to live without severe pain, and inability to participate, at least minimally, in human experience.

The first condition, recognizes the possibility that some infants may be born with irreparable lesions incompatible with life. While basic care should never be neglected for those already in the dying state, efforts aimed at prolonging life are best viewed as harming rather than helping such an infant.

The second condition envisions the case of an infant who is in constant severe pain that cannot be alleviated either by immediate or long-term treatment.

The third condition is perhaps the most controversial, and therefore needs some explanation. Judgment that an infant is unable to participate in human experience requires projection on the basis of indirect measurements. One must be able to say that there is no reasonable expectation that the infant will ever be able to respond affectively and cognitively to human attention and caring or to engage in communication with others. The criterion has to do with the presence or absence of capacity, not merely with degrees of deviation from the norm.

In applying this capacity criterion, we judge that the independent moral value of every infant requires cautious interpretation and that, in doubtful cases, it is better to err on the side of sustaining life. Thus a baby with Down's syndrome (mongoloidism), although sure to be mentally deficient, should be given life-sustaining therapy as a rule whenever needed; an anencephalic baby (born without a developed brain) should not be resuscitated or sustained.[5]

Some reasons for a conservative criterion. Some
may disagree with the conservative criterion proposed,
but a number of supporting reasons may be cited. First,
the moral value of the infant, regardless of its characteristics, exerts a strong demand for caution upon
those responsible for its well-being. Second, reaction
against the versatility with which medicine can preserve
life may lead to an overly broad definition of categories
of useless life, such as the senile, the costly, the
unattractive, the unproductive. These, some might say,
should be dispatched with easy conscience. We fear
that such a reaction would seriously damage the sensitivity to the value of human life that is essential to
civilization and to medicine as a humane art.

The principle also respects another important ethical stance, namely, protection of the most vulnerable.
We have chosen the conservative criterion in the hope
of steering a middle course between an undiscriminating
policy of saving and sustaining all life and inconsider-
ately consigning to destruction the most vulnerable.

Finally, diagnosis and prognosis are, by their very
nature, probabilistic judgments. It is extremely difficult to forecast the ability of an endangered infant
to participate in human experience; no single, clear
criterion is available. Even as medical experience
grows and skills improve, decisions will still be made
without absolute certainty about outcome. While the
moral certitude requisite for acting in good conscience
does not exclude the possibility of error, it does
require that judgments be based on reasonably strong
evidence and that one act cautiously in the face of
clear doubt. Thus, in questions of the survival of
endangered infants, the capacity prognosis criterion
should be applied with a bias favoring survival rather
than death.

Disagreements and the Quality of Life: The Seventh Proposition

This proposition concerns possible conflicts among the responsibility of the parents, the duty of the physician and the interest of the state. We urge a hierarchy of considerations, so that all decisions give first importance to the moral value of the infant. As principal bearers of the burden of defective children, parents deserve particular consideration but their interest is secondary to whatever can be determined about the best interests of the infant. It is important to note that physician advocacy for the infant should be understood as including, on some occasions, defense of the usefulness of continued therapy and, on others, recommending its termination when it appears that only harm (as defined above) would result from prolonging the infant's life.

The Relief of Pain and Euthanasia: The Eighth Proposition

The eighth proposition brings us into the euthanasia debate.[6] Some commentators call the withdrawal of life support technology, or the use of non-lethal (but probably life-shortening) doses of analgesics, "passive" or "indirect" euthanasia. In this context "active" euthanasia or "mercy killing" means taking some directly lethal action against the patient's life.[7]

Our position asserts that pain relief is part of good medical care of the dying and that the side effect of hastening death is compatible with both respect for the infant's moral value and the conscientious carrying out of the physician's duty.

The line drawn here between active and passive euthanasia is sometimes called a moral quibble.[8] Critics point out that in either case the infant dies and that the physician and/or parents choose the infant's death rather than his survival. With the end result

and the conscious choice the same, it seems irrational
to have scruples about the means, especially when it
can be argued that a speedier death is more merciful.[9]
These points are very persuasive.

However, several other considerations underly this
position. On pragmatic grounds, we note that in no
U.S. jurisdiction is mercy killing excepted from the
common law prohibition of murder.[10] Until statutes
legalizing mercy killing are on the books, a moral policy
endorsing active euthanasia is meaningless. We also
observe that many physicians perceive serving as the
agent of death as quite foreign to their role of providing terminal care and pain relief to a dying patient.[11]
An active euthanasia policy would have to designate an
appropriate executioner.[12]

Finally, as a general rule, the common good of
society and the rights of individuals seem best served
by reluctance to legitimize widespread authority to
terminate human life. This reluctance grows not from
a paranoid anticipation of extensive infanticide, but
from awareness that social practices tend to modify and
spread. There are a variety of life situations where
speedy death might appear to be a merciful solution to
real problems, e.g., severe mental deficiency, profound emotional disorders, and crippling old age. But,
in each of these situations, the active euthanasia
solution legitimizes a practice that is theoretically
difficult to contain.[13] Unless forms of due process
can be devised to contain the practice and give absolute
protection to the rights of all vulnerable, voiceless,
and "useless" members of society, it seems foolhardy
and dangerous to urge a policy of active euthanasia
for dying neonates.

Allocation of Limited Resources:
The Ninth Proposition

This proposition deals with allocation of limited
medical resources as the question arises in the intensive

care nursery. Up to this point, moral considerations have focused on the well-being of the individual infant. Now, a new element is introduced, i.e., the comparison of need between two individuals. It becomes difficult to apply the rule "Do no harm," since either decision may effect some harm without providing a compensatory benefit to the one harmed.

The rule of triage. This dilemma may be illuminated by the traditional medico-moral rule of triage, whereby casualties in military and civil disasters are typically divided into three groups: (1) those who will not survive even if treated, (2) those who will survive without treatment, and (3) the priority group of those who need treatment in order to survive. A further triage among the priority group can give preference to those who can be reactivated quickly, or who hold crucial positions of responsibility. Considerations of the common good become relevant in such decisions.

Similarly, in the selection of infants to receive various kinds of treatment, the interest of the state can be invoked as an ethical consideration since the state has an interest in the recognition of values, in fulfillment of responsibilities and duties, in the fair and efficient distribution of benefits, and in the promotion of the population's health. These interests are directed toward a common good which, in a situation such as this, may be the predominant consideration. Because it is impossible to treat all infants in need, preference should be given those with the greatest hope of surviving with maximal function.

Some hazards. The use of this principle must be approached with gravity and caution. First, what appear to be considerations of the common good are in practice often special interest considerations in disguise. Those identified with certain persons or classes may see their favored treatment as contributing to the common good. Second, the hope of survival with maximal function is predicated not only on the infant's physical potential, but also on the nature of the socioeconomic world it enters. Thus, estimates of the quality of future care may affect its selection for continued intensive care. Third, selection of better-prognosis infants could be strongly motivated more by the physician's interest in compiling favorable statistics, or in making quicker decisions, than the condition of one or more infants might warrant. Thus, the principle of neonatal triage, while instructive in general, risks serious bias.[14]

PROCEDURAL RECOMMENDATIONS

A moral policy should include both ethical propositions (see above) and procedural recommendations for institutional and social arrangements that will aid deliberation, decision and action based on those propositions. We have discussed ethical propositions in terms of micro-decisions to be made by persons who bear responsibilities and duties in regard to particular infants at risk, but the discussion of recommendations deals with macro-decisions where issues of state interest, social costs, and economic considerations come to the fore in the complex sphere of public policy.

The following recommendations are offered more as a schema for further inquiry than as a thoroughly worked-out policy position.

1. Research in neonatology should be coordinated at the national level in the interest of both efficiency and caution.

2. Neonatal intensive care should be so organized on a regional basis that quality and access are relatively equal among various communities, continuing information on techniques can be shared, and adequate epidemiological data can be gathered and compared.

3. On the basis of clinical experience, professionals in neonatal intensive care should refine clinical criteria that specify the conditions under which life can be prolonged without pain and with the potential

for human experience. These criteria should be communicated broadly within the pediatric, obstetric, and mental health community.

4. Resuscitation criteria should be established with full awareness of the economic and medical implications of providing this care. Estimates should be made of the financial cost to society of prolonging life at a humane level depending upon the condition at birth.

5. Delivery room policy, based on certain criteria, should state conditions in which resuscitation will not be attempted. Such policies should be openly communicated to health professionals and prospective parents.

6. Prospective parents should be made aware of the problems associated with neonatal intensive care. Explanatory and supportive counselling of parents should be a mandatory component of medical care involving endangered neonates. While recognizing that parents often will be unable or unwilling to make decisions, medical professionals should always accept the principle that the responsibility should if possible be borne by the parents, and attempt to help but not force them to make the decision.

7. The decision to terminate care for an infant requires sufficient time for observation, mature assessment, and parental involvement in the decision. Thus, it is more ethical, although perhaps more agonizing, to terminate care after a period of time than to withhold resuscitative measures at the moment of birth. This time element should be included in an accepted and publicly acknowledged policy in pediatric and obstetric practice.

8. Regional neonatal intensive care units should establish advisory boards consisting of health professionals and other involved and interested persons. Such boards should not be charged with particular decisions about specific infants; this remains the responsibility of the parents with advice and concurrence of the physician. The boards would discuss the problems of the

unit and make a periodic retrospective review of the difficult decisions. They would assess the criteria for diagnosis and prognosis in terms of medical validity and social acceptability. By bringing together a variety of experience, belief and attitude, they would provide a wider human environment for decisionmaking than might otherwise be available. To implement such a procedure, a neonatal intensive care unit could review its experience prospectively for each case in which a decision had to be made. All pertinent data could be recorded in a case summary, which would be reviewed monthly, would describe the current process of ethical decisionmaking in the unit, and provide a basis for any changes that might be planned.

9. Some infants may be abandoned by their parents or, because of their conditions, be maintained in an institution for long periods or for life. Accordingly neonatology must concern itself with the adequacy of such institutions. Those advocating maximum use of intensive care must also advocate the development of humane continuing care facilities, as well as adequate funding of programs to assist families with children needing special attention at home or in institutions. Thus neonatology must take into account the continuing specialized care that will be needed by each of those individuals who survive life-threatening neonatal disorders with the aid of intensive care therapy.

CONCLUSION

In the neonatal intensive care situation some people must try to act in the best interests of others who cannot speak for themselves. To assess rationally such situations is an important contribution to the work of safeguarding the rights of these infants. We do not presume to have spoken the final word, but have espoused a definite position in order to invite reflection and debate. We hope this effort will promote more sensitive appreciation of the needs and rights of all the participants in the drama of newborn intensive care.

NOTES

NOTES TO INTRODUCTION--JONSEN

[1]The conference was jointly sponsored by the Health
Policy Program and the Department of Pediatrics of the
University of California, San Francisco, and supported
by funds from the Robert Wood Johnson Foundation. The
conference was directed by William H. Tooley, M.D. and
Roderic H. Phibbs, M.D., neonatologists working in the
Intensive Care Nursery, Moffitt Hospital, University of
California, San Francisco (hereafter UCSF) and Albert
R. Jonsen, Ph.D., Associate Professor of Bioethics,
School of Medicine (UCSF). Michael J. Garland, Ph.D.,
Lecturer in Bioethics, School of Medicine (UCSF), served
as conference coordinator.

Conference participants included: Eileen Brewer,
M.D., pediatrician (UCSF); John Clausen, Ph.D., sociol-
ogist, University of California, Berkeley (hereafter
UCB); Danner Clouser, Ph.D., philosopher, Hershey Medical
Center (HMC), Pennsylvania State University; Marianna
Cohen, M.S.W., social worker (UCSF); Robert K. Creasy,
M.D., obstetrician (UCSF); Morris Davis, J.D., M.P.H.,
editor, *Masks, Journal of Black Health Perspectives*;
Jane Hunt, Ph.D., research psychologist (UCB); Robert
Jaffe, M.D., obstetrician (UCSF); Marcia Kramer, Ph.D.,
economist, State University of New York, Stony Brook;
Alan Margolis, M.D., obstetrician (UCSF); F. Raymond
Marks, J.D., attorney, Childhood and Government Project
(UCB); Laura Nader, Ph.D., anthropologist (UCB); Nicholas
Nelson, M.D., pediatrician (HMC); David Perlman, science
editor, San Francisco *Chronicle*; Teresa Poirier, R.N.
(UCSF); Gloria Powell, M.D., psychiatrist, University
of California, Los Angeles; Clement A. Smith, M.D.,
pediatrician, Harvard Medical School.

Additional material was contributed to this volume
by Philip R. Lee, M.D., internist, Professor of Community
Medicine and Director, Health Policy Program, School of

Notes to pp. 3 to 13

Medicine (UCSF); Diane Dooley, pre-doctoral Fellow, Health Policy Program, School of Medicine (UCSF); and Alex Stalcup, M.D., then Chief Resident, Pediatrics Service, Moffitt Hospital (UCSF).

[2]"The Problem and Its Limits: Relationship to Pediatrics," *Report of the Sixty-Fifth Ross Conference on Pediatric Research: Ethical Dilemmas in Current Obstetric and Newborn Care* (Columbus, Ohio: Ross Laboratories, 1973), p. 17.

[3]See F. Raymond Marks's paper below, especially p. 100 ff.

[4]See Marcia Kramer's paper below, pp. 75-93.

[5]See Jane Hunt's paper below, especially pp. 45-49.

[6]See below, pp. 142-155.

[7]See Marianna Cohen's discussion of parental participation in these decisions, below, pp. 54-63.

NOTES TO TOOLEY AND PHIBBS PAPER

[1]Cecil M. Drillien, *The Growth and Development of the Prematurely Born Infant* (Baltimore: Williams and Wilkins Co., 1964).

[2]L. O. Lubchenco, M. Delivoria-Papadopoulos and D. Searls, "Long-term follow-up studies of prematurely born infants. II. Influence of birthweight and gestational age on sequelae," *Journal of Pediatrics,* 80(3):509-512 (March 1972).

Notes to pp. 13 to 16

[3]Robert O. Fisch, Howard J. Gravem and Rolf R.
Engel, "Neurological status of survivors of neonatal
respiratory distress syndrome," *Journal of Pediatrics*,
73 (3): 395-403 (September 1968).

[4]Mildred T. Stahlman, "What Evidence Exists That
Intensive Care Has Changed the Incidence of Intact Sur-
vival," *Report of the Fifty-Ninth Ross Conference on
Pediatric Research: Problems of Neonatal Intensive Care
Units*, ed. J. L. Lucey (Columbus, Ohio: Ross Labora-
tories, 1969), pp. 17-24.

[5]L. O. Lubchenco, et al., "Newborn Intensive Care
and Long-term Prognosis," *Developmental Medicine and
Child Neurology*, 16(4):421-431 (August 1974).

[6]Ann L. Stewart and E. O. R. Reynolds, "Improved
Prognosis for Infants of Very Low Birthweight," *Pediatrics*, 54(6):724-735 (December 1974).

[7]P. M. Fitzhardinge and M. Ramsay, "The Improving
Outlook for the Small Prematurely Born Infant," *Develop-
mental Medicine and Child Neurology*, 15(4):447-459
(August 1973).

NOTES TO PANEL DISCUSSION

[1]Alex Stalcup, M.D., Chief Resident, Pediatrics
Service, moderated the discussion, with a panel that included Leslie Carey, R.N., Senior Staff Nurse, Intensive
Care Nursery; Michael Siegel, M.D., Senior Pediatric
Resident; Eileen Ziomek, M.D., Intern (all of UCSF); and
Martin Cohen, M.D., Chief Pediatric Resident, San Francisco General Hospital. This presentation was planned
and organized by Drs. Stalcup and William H. Tooley, and
Professor Albert R. Jonsen, all of UCSF; the transcript
was edited by Anne M. Schmid, editor for the Department
of Pediatrics.

Notes to pp. 16 to 20

 The cases discussed here are composed of elements from real situations in order to make them representative of experiences in intensive care nurseries throughout the country. The same cases were discussed at the Sonoma Conference, where several papers in this volume were originally presented.

 [2]The Apgar score is a quick test used by physicians to determine the degree of asphyxiation of a baby at birth. It consists of rating the baby on a scale of 0-2 in each of five categories as indicated in the following chart. The ratings are totaled to give the score. A score of 0-2 indicates asphyxiation requiring emergency resuscitation. A score of 3-6 indicates mild asphyxiation usually responsive to suctioning of the airway and brief ventilation with oxygen mask and pressure bag. The infant with a score of 7 or more rarely needs any resuscitation.

APGAR SCORE

SIGN	SCORE		
	0	1	2
Heart rate	Absent	Below 100	Over 100
Respiratory effort	Absent	Weak, irregular	Good, crying
Muscle tone	Flaccid	Some flexion of extremities	Well flexed
Reflex irritability (catheter in nose)	No response	Grimace	Cough or sneeze
Color	Blue, pale	Body pink, extremities blue	Completely pink

Notes to pp. 34 to 39

NOTES TO SMITH PAPER

[1]Harry S. Dweck, et al., "Early Development of the Tiny Premature Infant," *American Jouranl of Diseases of Children*, 126 (1):28-34 (July 1973).

[2]Robert H. Usher, Royal Victoria Hospital, Montreal: personal communication.

[3]L. S. Prod'hom, et al., "Care of the Seriously Ill Neonate with Hyaline Membrane Disease and with Sepsis (Sclerema Neonatorum)," *Pediatrics*, 53 (2): 170-181 (February 1974).

[4]Raymond S. Duff and A. G. M. Campbell, "Moral and Ethical Dilemmas in the Special-Care Nursery," *New England Journal of Medicine*, 289 (17): 890-894 (October 25, 1973). See p. 891.

NOTES TO HUNT PAPER

[1]Cf. Cecil M. Drillien, "Aetiology and Outcome in Low-birthweight Infants," *Developmental Medicine and Child Neurology*, 14(5):563-574 (October 1972); L. O. Lubchenco, et al., "Newborn Intensive Care and Long-term Prognosis," *Developmental Medicine and Child Neurology*, 16(4):421-431 (August 1974); Mildred Stahlman, et al., "A Six-Year Follow-Up of Clinical Hyaline Membrane Disease," *Pediatrics Clinics of North America*, 20(2): 433-446 (May 1973); E. W. Outerbridge, M. Ramsay and L. Stern, "Developmental Follow-up of Survivors of Neonatal Respiratory Failure," *Critical Care Medicine,* 2(12): 23-27 (January-February 1974).

[2]Cf. L. O. Lubchenco, note 1 above; P. M. Fitzhardinge and M. Ramsay, "The Improving Outlook for the Small Prematurely Born Infant," *Developmental Medicine and Child Neurology*, 15(4):447-459 (August 1973).

Notes to pp. 40 to 47

³Cf. L. O. Lubchenco, et al., note 1 above; P. M. Fitzhardinge and M. Ramsay, note 2 above; Harry S. Dweck, et al., "Early Development of the Tiny Premature Infant," *American Journal of Diseases of Children*, 126 (1):28-34 (July 1973).

⁴Jane V. Hunt, William H. Tooley, et al., "Mental Development of Children with Birthweights < 1500 G.," abstract of paper in *Clinical Research*, 22(2):240-A (February 1974).

⁵Roderic H. Phibbs, William H. Tooley, et al., "Development of Children Who Had Received Intra-Uterine Transfusions," *Pediatrics*, 47(4):689-697 (April 1971).

⁶See E. W. Outerbridge, note 1 above. See also R. Dinwiddie, et al., "Quality of Survival after Artificial Ventilation of the Newborn," *Archives of Disease in Childhood*, 49(9):703-710 (September 1974).

⁷Jane V. Hunt, "Environmental Risk in Fetal and Neonatal Life and Measured Infant Intelligence," in M. Lewis, ed., *Origins of Intelligence* (New York: Plenum Press, 1975), pp. 223-258.

⁸F. Cukier, C. Amiel-Tison, and A. Minkowski, "Hyaline Membrane Disease in Neonates Treated with Artificial Ventilation: Neurological and Intellectual Sequelae at Two to Five Years of Age," *Critical Care Medicine*, 2(5):265-269 (September-October 1974).

⁹Ralph Reitan and Thomas J. Boll, "Neuropsychological Correlates of Minimal Brain Dysfunction," *Annals of the New York Academy of Sciences*, 205:65-88 (February 1973).

Notes to pp. 47 to 55

[10]Cecil M. Drillien, "Longitudinal Study of the Growth and Development of Prematurely Born Children. Part VII: Mental Development 2-5 Years," *Archives of Disease in Childhood*, 36(187):233-240 (June 1961); H. Knobloch and B. Pasamanick, "Predicting Intellectual Potential in Infancy: Some Variables Affecting Validity of Developmental Diagnosis," *American Journal of Diseases of Children*, 106(1):43-51 (July 1963).

[11]Cf. Rick Heber and Howard Garber, *An Experiment in the Prevention of Cultural-Familial Mental Retardation* (Washington, D.C.: 1970). Sponsored by the U.S. Department of Health, Education, and Welfare, Rehabilitation Services Administration.

For additional references, see also: Cecil M. Drillien, *The Growth and Development of the Prematurely Born Infant* (Baltimore: Williams and Wilkins Co., 1964); L. O. Lubchenco, Frederick Horner, Linda H. Reed, et al., "Sequelae of Premature Birth: Evaluation of Premature Infants of Low Birth Weights at Ten Years of Age," *American Journal of Diseases of Children*, 106(1): 101-115 (July 1963); Nancy Bayley et al., "Environmental Factors in the Development of Institutionalized Children," in Jerome Helmuth, ed., *Exceptional Infant: Studies in Abnormalities*, Vol. 2 (New York: Brunner/ Mazel, 1971). See pp. 450-472.

NOTES TO COHEN PAPER

[1]Erich Lindemann, "Symptomatology and Management of Acute Grief," *American Journal of Psychiatry*, 101 (2):141-148 (September 1944); Audrey T. McCollom and Herbert A. Schwartz, "Social Work and the Mourning Parent," *Social Work*, 17(1):25-36 (January 1972); Lydia Rapoport, "The State of Crisis: Some Theoretical Considerations," *Social Service Review*, 36(2):211-217 (June 1962).

Notes to pp. 58 to 68

[2]David M. Kaplan and Edward A. Mason, "Maternal
Reactions to Premature Birth Viewed as an Acute Emotional Disorder," *American Journal of Orthopsychiatry*,
30(3):539-552 (July 1960).

[3]John H. Kennell and Marshall H. Klaus, "Care of
the Mother of the High-Risk Infant," *Clinical Obstetrics
and Gynecology*, 14(3):926-954 (September 1971).

NOTES TO LEE AND DOOLEY PAPER

[1]U.S., Department of Health, Education, and Welfare,
Maternal and Child Health Service, *Children Who Received
Physicians' Services Under the Crippled Children's Program. Fiscal Year 1971* (Rockville, Maryland: Department of Health, Education, and Welfare, 1973), Table 16.

[2]U.S., Congress, House of Representatives, Committee
on Ways and Means, *National Health Insurance Resource
Book* (Washington, D.C.: 1974), p. 498.

[3]U.S., Department of Health, Education, and Welfare,
Maternal and Child Health Service, *Children Served in
Mental Retardation Clinics, Fiscal Years 1970-1972*
(Washington, D.C.: 1973), p. 1.

[4]James S. Kakalik, et al., *Services for Handicapped
Youth: A Program Overview* (prepared for the U.S. Depart-
ment of Health, Education, and Welfare) (Santa Monica,
California: Rand Corporation, May 1973), pp. 175, 234.

[5]Children's Defense Fund, *Children Out of School
in America* (Cambridge, Massachusetts: 1974), p. 94.

[6]Kakalik, note 4 above, p. 89.

Notes to pp. 68 to 76

[7] Robert Morris, "Welfare Reform 1973: The Social Services Dimension," *Science*, 181(4099):515-522 (August 10, 1973).

[8] Executive Office of the President, Office of Management and Budget, *Special Analyses: Budget of the United States Government Fiscal Year 1976* (Washington, D.C.: 1975), p. 184.

[9] Ruth Roemer, et al., *Planning Urban Health Services from Jungle to System* (New York: Springer Publishing Co., Inc., 1975).

[10] Morris, note 7 above, p. 516.

[11] Kakalik, note 4 above, p. 190.

[12] Karen Davis, "A Decade of Policy Developments in Providing Care for Low-Income Families" (Unpublished manuscript, 1975), pp. 9, 10.

[13] George A. Silver, "Impact of Child Health Legislation in the State of Connecticut" (Unpublished manuscript, 1974), p. 25.

[14] Kakalik, note 4 above, p. 92.

[15] Silver, note 13 above, p. 15.

NOTES TO KRAMER PAPER

[1] The interested reader will find a wealth of intriguing material in the growing economic literature dealing with fertility, crime, discrimination, marriage, product safety, education and the environment.

Notes to pp. 76 to 78

[2]This was strikingly evident at the Sonoma conference: in specifying the various conditions under which
a decision to withhold or withdraw intensive care ever
could be morally justified, the non-economists were unanimous in their omission of the economic factor. For
some, this may have been an oversight or an assumption
that the response need only be applicable to urban,
middle class America in the 1970's, but beyond this it
would seem to reflect a strongly held conviction that
costs *should not* count.

[3]It is not only in poor societies that the provision
of costly NIC to some could jeopardize other lives. In
wartime or other emergencies, even the richest communities may experience an acute scarcity of medical personnel and/or facilities. In "normal" times, there is
even the grotesque possibility—instances were documented
at the Sonoma conference—that all intensive care units
may be in use when a newly eligible baby is born. Here,
the real cost of saving one infant may well be the death
of another.

[4]In India, for example, the birth rate in 1973 was
42 per 1,000 population and the infant mortality rate
139 per 1,000 births. Conservatively estimating infant
morbidity at twice the level of infant mortality, that
means that 1.2 percent of the population would be eligible for NIC each year (.042 x .139 x 2 x 100). If NIC
hospitalization costs were $4,000 per patient (about
1/3 of the U.S. level, as data below indicate) they
would amount to $24 per capita per year, or 22 percent
of the $110 per capita gross national product. (Data
are from Population Reference Bureau, Inc., *1973 World
Population Data Sheet*, Washington, D.C.).

[5]"The Specter of Eugenics," *Commentary*, 57:25-33
(March 1974). See p. 32.

Notes to pp. 80 to 85

[6]Richard Hatwick, "Economics and the Impact on Society," *Report of the Sixty-Fifth Ross Conference on Pediatric Research: Ethical Dilemmas in Current Obstetric and Newborn Care* (Columbus, Ohio: Ross Laboratories, 1973), pp. 41-43.

[7]Ritchie H. Reed and Susan McIntosh, "Costs of Children," in Elliott R. Morss and Ritchie H. Reed, eds., *Economic Aspects of Population Change*, Vol. 2, Research Reports, The Commission on Population Growth and the American Future (Washington, D.C.: 1972), pp. 333-350. See p. 345.

[8]Since parents generally do not anticipate "capturing" the adult earnings of their offspring, the $98,000 represents the sum they are demonstrably willing and able to spend to raise a normal first child.

[9]Ronald W. Conley, *The Economics of Mental Retardation* (Baltimore: Johns Hopkins University Press, 1973), p. 298.

[10]$16,347 (for NIC) + ($3,450 + $1,173) (70 years) + $2,500 (20 years) = $389,957. $16,347 was the average NIC cost in 1973 for all UCSF babies with birth weight under 1500 grams who survived (Table 1). The assumption of a normal lifespan for the abnormal survivors is not intended to be typical. Extraordinary medical expenses are omitted from this computation.

[11]Conley, note 9 above, p. 96.

[12]My thanks to Marianna Cohen for pointing out the possibility of there being a cost saving associated with NIC.

Notes to pp. 87 to 100

[13] For simplicity, the present illustration refers exclusively to dollar costs and benefits. A full accounting would of course also strive to take account of the intangible, non-monetary costs and benefits imposed upon society by individuals (e.g., congestion and pollution in the cost column, parental satisfaction in the benefit category).

[14] For example, if N = $30,000 and (C-B) = -$100,000 for the former child, net incremental cost to society is -$70,000 before discounting (i.e., a cost saving) but is possibly +$20,000 after discounting if the benefits are far off and the discount rate high. In contrast, if N = $2,000 and (C-B) = $100,000 for the latter child, the net incremental cost is $102,000 before discounting but possibly only $12,000 after it. (Each case assumes that the present value of the future $100,000 is $10,000).

[15] Conley, note 9 above, p. 96.

[16] The range of possibilities is infinite, since any of the three possible outcomes can be assigned the "moral weight" of 1, and weights for each of the remaining two outcomes can range from 0 to 1, inclusive.

NOTES TO MARKS PAPER

[1] 410 U.S. 113 (1973).

[2] *Death at an Early Age* (Boston: Houghton-Mifflin, 1967).

[3] In some ways, with respect to babies not heretofore viable, the medical profession is in the position

Notes to pp. 100 to 104

of the Good Samaritan. There may be a requirement that once intervention has occurred, there is an obligation to see the process through to an acceptable end.

[4] *Gleitman v. Cosgrove*, 227 A.2d 689 (New Jersey, 1967). A dissenter in this case did introduce into his opinion a gradient between life itself and quality of life.

[5] *Zapeda v. Zapeda*, 190 N.E. 2d 849 (Ill. App., 1963).

[6] *Williams v. State of New York*, 260 N.Y.S. 2d 953 (1965).

[7] See Sir Henry Maine, *Ancient Law* (London: Oxford University Press, 1959); first published 1861.

[8] See, for example, the discussion in Anthony Shaw, "Dilemmas of 'Informed Consent' in Children," *New England Journal of Medicine*, 289(17):885-890 (October 25, 1973).

[9] It may be that legislative or judicial adoptions of fictions may occur, at some point, for "non-human" human babies.

[10] See Ludwig Edelstein, *The Hippocratic Oath* (Baltimore: Johns Hopkins University Press, 1943), p. 10.

[11] See Guido Calabresi, "Reflections on Medical Experimentation in Humans," *Daedalus*, 98(2):387-405 (1969). Also Calabresi, *The Costs of Accidents: A Legal and Economic Analysis* (New Haven: Yale University Press, 1970).

Notes to pp. 104 to 107

[12]Problems arise even where we don't know the name, if we have reason to believe that the selection process will be class biased rather than democratic or random. Highway deaths are democratic--the automobile is the great equalizer. War deaths, however, frequently cause us problems if the method of selecting those to be risked is biased. What about neonatal deaths? What about the lives of those spared by the new technology? Are they closer to random than not?

[13]"Attitudes Toward Defective Newborns," *The Hastings Center Studies*, 2(1):21-32 (January 1974).

[14]Ibid., p. 27. See also Philippe Aries, *Centuries of Childhood* (New York: Knopf, 1962). Aries suggests that the industrial revolution changed expectations of children. In a previous work, the principal author of the present article suggests that after the industrial revolution--at least in this country--it was not religion that became the opiate of the masses, it was children. See "Detours on the Road to Maturity: A View of the Legal Conception of Growing Up and Letting Go," *39 Law and Contemporary Problems*, 3:78-92 (Summer 1975).

[15]"How Much Do We Want to Know About the Unborn? Amniocentesis may force us to make choices we wish we didn't have," *The Hastings Center Report*, 3(1):8-9 (February 1973).

[16]California Civil Code, Title 2, Chap. 2, Sec. 227b.

[17]See Anthony Shaw, note 8 above and, in the same publication, Raymond S. Duff and A.G.M. Campbell, "Moral and Ethical Dilemmas in the Special-Care Nursery," 890-894. See also the *Report of the Sixty-Fifth Ross Conference on Pediatric Research: Ethical Dilemmas in Current Obstetric and Newborn Care* (1973); H. Tristram

Notes to pp. 107 to 122

Engelhardt, Jr., "Euthanasia and Children: The Injury of Continued Existence," in "Letters to the Editor," *The Journal of Pediatrics*, 83(1):170-171 (July 1973).

[18]See, for example, California Welfare and Institutions Code, Sec. 7275.

[19]Ross Conference, see note 17 above, p. 81 et seq.

[20]See Joseph Fletcher, "Indicators of Humanhood: A Tentative Profile of Man," *The Hastings Center Report*, 2(5) (November 1972).

[21]The non-distinct interests last well beyond infancy. See *Wisconsin v. Yoder*, 406 U.S. 205 (1972), where the issue of whether Amish children could be exempted from high school was treated as a conflict between parents and the state, and not an issue about which a child could evidence a distinct wish. Mr. Justice Douglas, dissenting, asked: "Why not ask the children?"

[22]See, for example, *In re Sampson*, 317 N.Y.S. 2d 641 (New York, 1970).

[23]Informed consent is discussed under Question IV, p. 120 ff.

[24]See Eleanor S. Glass, "Restructuring Informed Consent: Legal Therapy for the Doctor-Patient Relationship," 79 *Yale Law Journal* 8:1533-1576 (1970); Jon R. Waltz and Thomas W. Scheuneman, "Informed Consent to Therapy," 64 *Northwestern University Law Review* 5:628-650 (1970).

172

Notes to pp. 123 to 136

[25]Sir Henry Maine, note 7 above, observed the trends in developments of several societies. He noted that as a society was most primitive, it relied heavily on mystery and fictions, hiding from itself the bases of action. As society matured more, there was an emergence of equity--an open interference with a rule of law in the name of mercy and out of consideration for the particular acts and actors. Finally, when a society matured, it relied on legislation more and more, and on open statement of the premises of rules and actions. In the nursery, now, we are somewhere between fiction and equity.

[26]See R. H. Mnookin, "Foster Care--In Whose Best Interest?" *Harvard Education Review*, 43(4):599-638 (1973).

NOTES TO GARLAND PAPER

[1]*Philosophy and Public Affairs*, 2(1):37-65 (Fall 1972).

[2]*The Hastings Center Studies*, 2(2):37-46 (May 1974).

[3]*Perspectives in Biology and Medicine*, 16(4):529-557 (Summer 1973).

[4]*Journal of the American Medical Association*, 229 (2):172-176 (July 8, 1974).

[5]*New England Journal of Medicine*, 292(2):75-78 (January 9, 1975).

[6]"Abortion," *The Thomist*, 37:174-226 (1973). See also "Feticide/Infanticide Upon Request," *Religion and Life*, 39:170-186 (1970).

Notes to pp. 136 to 148

[7] *The Ethics of Genetic Control* (Garden City, New York: Anchor Press/Doubleday, 1974), pp. 132-143, 185-186.

[8] *Beneficent Euthanasia*, ed. Marvin Kohl (Buffalo, New York: Prometheus Books, 1975).

NOTES TO JONSEN AND GARLAND PAPER

[1] Daniel J. Callahan, *Abortion: Law, Choice and Morality* (New York: Collier/Macmillan, 1970), p. 341.

[2] Nurses also have a special professional relationship to the infant, the parents, and physicians in the provision of intensive care. Their role in decisions about continuation of therapy for endangered infants merits full discussion and articulation with an understanding of the roles of physicians and parents. Other, non-medical, persons such as social workers and clergy, also play important roles in the decisionmaking process; these become apparent when one focuses on the decision process itself. For the present discussion we have set aside these other considerations in order to focus directly on the parent-physician relationship.

[3] The word *state* is used here to refer both to society as a whole and to the legitimate institutional structures that control and distribute goods and services through legislative, administrative, and judicial functions.

[4] B. Gert, *The Moral Rules* (New York: Harper and Row, 1966) pp. 60, 104.

[5] James M. Gustafson, "Mongolism, Parental Desires and the Right to Life," *Perspectives in Biology and Medicine*, 16(4):529-557 (Summer 1973).

Notes to pp. 150 to 151

[6]See, for example: J. Bennett, "Whatever the Consequences," *Analysis* 26:82 (1966); P. Foot, "The Problem of Abortion and the Doctrine of the Double Effect," *Oxford Review*, 5:5 (1967); R. A. McCormick, *Ambiguity in Moral Choice* (Milwaukee: Marquette University Press, 1973); and the following from *BioScience*, 23(8) (August 1973): Sissela Bok, "Euthanasia and the Care of the Dying," 461-466; David W. Meyers, "The Legal Aspects of Medical Euthanasia, " 467-470; Diana Crane, "Physicians' Attitudes Toward the Treatment of Critically Ill Patients," 471-474; and Eric J. Cassell, "Permission to Die," 475-478.

[7]James Rachels, "Active and Passive Euthanasia," *New England Journal of Medicine*, 292(2):78-80 (January 9, 1975).

[8]Beverly Kelsey, "Which Infants Shall Live? Who Should Decide? An interview with Dr. Raymond S. Duff," *The Hastings Center Report*, 5(2):5-8 (April 1975). See p. 7.

[9]Joseph Fletcher, "Ethics and Euthanasia," *American Journal of Nursing*, 73(4):670-675 (April 1973).

[10]Meyers, note 6 above.

[11]See letters under title "Euthanasia" in *New England Journal of Medicine*, 292(16):863 (April 17, 1975).

[12]To the question, "Would it ever be right to intervene directly to kill a self-sustaining infant (in cases where the decision has been made to let the baby die)?" A neonatologist gave the following loaded response: "Yes, if the parents administered the syringe of KCl prepared by the judge, and all the lawyers,

Notes to pp. 151 to 153

priests, economists, psychologists, and journalists within a 50 mile radius were witnesses and no physicians,
nurses, or medical or nursing students were allowed to
be present." (See also App. Question 3.)

[13]Leo Alexander, "Medical Science Under Dictator-
ship," *New England Journal of Medicine*, 241(2):39-47
(July 14, 1949).

[14]Jane Hunt, in a personal communication, regis-
tered vigorous opposition to this proposition. "I maintain...(neonatal triage) turns out *not* to be a proper
ethical question because there is *no* ethical solution.
One rule is as good as another, unlike the military
triage. You can never articulate a policy which sepa-
rates 'common good' from 'special interest' because the
latter can be put forward as cogent arguments for the
former. For example, consider the comparison between
the wanted and the unwanted infant." (See also her
paper in this volume, pp. 39-53.)

APPENDIX

Four Critical Questions

The 20 participants at the Sonoma Conference on
Ethical Issues in Neonatal Intensive Care prepared answers to four clinical-ethical questions. The following tables--one for each question--collate their responses with respect to the points of reference that define particular positions. This presentation sacrifices
the internal consistency of individual answers in the
interest of displaying a spectrum of reference points
for the problems considered.

Each table presents five categories, with the
first three referring directly to the infant's condition:
general physical status, *general "human" status*, and
medical indications. The other two categories refer to
conditions external to the individual infant: *family
situation* and *miscellaneous conditions* (e.g., review
and consultation procedures, informed consent.)

The questions address the issues of initial intervention, withdrawal of life support already initiated,
active lethal intervention, and allocation of the limited resources of a neonatal intensive care unit.

Re: Question #1

Many infants are born in need of vigorous resuscitation. The decision whether or not to treat them must
be made immediately. Given a situation where such

therapy is readily available, "Would It Ever Be Right Not To Resuscitate an Infant at Birth?"

Re: Question #2

Many infants who are candidates for intensive care therapy at birth have underlying anomalies, lesions, or disease states that are not readily apparent when the decision to initiate therapy is made. Further, in the course of therapy, complications sometimes develop that result in severe neurological damage. Given the situation of an infant who is receiving intensive care but who has a clearly recognized defect, "Would It Ever Be Right To Withdraw Life Support From a Clearly Diagnosed, Poor Prognosis Infant?"

Re: Question #3

Assuming that on the basis of a clear diagnosis and poor prognosis, a decision is made to let a given infant die, and further that the infant is now, and will be self-sustaining for some time, "Would It Ever Be Right To Intervene Directly To Kill a Self-Sustaining Infant?" (Insofar as distinction between active and passive euthanasia is valid, this question concerns active euthanasia, i.e., taking some directly lethal action against the life of the infant.)

Re: Question #4

When an infant is born who needs intensive care, an intensive care nursery may have no more room and no equivalent facilities may be available within a reasonable distance. If one of the infants already receiving intensive care is clearly diagnosed and has a poor prognosis, and the newcomer infant is judged with reasonable certitude to have a better prognosis, "Would It Ever Be Right To Displace Poor Prognosis Infant A in Order To Provide Intensive Care to Better Prognosis Infant B?"

All conditions have been given equal weight, phrased as if they were qualifying a "yes" response. All the participants answered "yes" to questions one and two, and nearly everyone answered "yes" to questions three and four. Where the answers were "no" or "uncertain", the reasons for these appear in footnotes.

QUESTION #1:   WOULD IT EVER BE RIGHT NOT TO RESUSCITATE
AN INFANT AT BIRTH?

ANSWERS: YES (unanimous) *(further comments listed
below under Limiting Conditions)*

LIMITING CONDITIONS: CHILD'S SITUATION

General Physical Status

1. If baby is dying (or is "dead") and there is no
hope of correcting the present lethal condition or
foreseeable related complications so that, if resuscitated, the baby would probably die in infancy

2. If baby is in pain which resuscitation will only
prolong

General "Human" Status

1. If the quality of life is and will be intolerable
as judged by most reasonable persons (the infant's
life will predictably involve greater suffering than
happiness and it will probably be without self-awareness or socializing capacities)

2. If the infant has no chance (or small chance) of
normal life

3. If the infant is clearly below human standards
for meaningful life

Medical Indications

1. If the infant is anencephalic

2. If the infant has severe central nervous system
disorders

Question 1 cont'd

3. If the infant has gross physical anomalies (e.g., no limbs)

4. If the infant has a (large) meningomyelocele

5. If the infant has Down's syndrome (and other chromosomal abnormalities)

6. If the infant is extremely premature or has an extremely low birthweight. (three cut-off lines proposed: (1) 900 grams; (2) 750 grams or 26 weeks gestation; (3) 500 grams or 22 weeks gestation)

7. If the infant has (major) hydrocephaly

8. If there has been a catastrophe in the birth canal

9. If the infant is porencephalic

10. If there is multiple absence of sense organs

11. If the infant is dead as evidenced by tissue decay

12. If there has been no fetal heartbeat for more than five minutes before birth

LIMITING CONDITIONS: FAMILY SITUATION

(Note: All conditions listed here presuppose that the infant is severely defective)

1. If the death of the infant would minimize the suffering of the parents

2. If the death of the infant would avoid unbearable financial costs to the family

3. If the death of the infant would avoid emotional burden to its siblings

4. If the parents already have a defective child

Question 1 cont'd

LIMITING CONDITIONS: MISCELLANEOUS

(Note: All conditions listed here presuppose that the infant is severely defective)

1.   If, insofar as possible, the parents participate in the decision

2.   If there is an open and consistent delivery room policy about nonresuscitation

3.   If there is prior informed consent from parents not to resuscitate under specific conditions

4.   If delivery room policy not to resuscitate is kept flexible in response to the state of the art

5.   If, insofar as possible, an advocate for the infant assists in the decision whether to resuscitate

6.   If costs to the state of infant's survival are considered

7.   If, in cases where gross and obvious structural anomalies are not present, decisions not to resuscitate would be reviewed by a board of physicians and others

QUESTION #2: WOULD IT EVER BE RIGHT TO WITHDRAW LIFE SUPPORT FROM A CLEARLY DIAGNOSED, POOR PROGNOSIS INFANT?

ANSWERS: YES (unanimous) *(further comments listed below under Limiting Conditions)*

LIMITING CONDITIONS: CHILD'S SITUATION

General Physical Status

1. If the infant is diagnosable as having gross defects (coupled with item 2 or 3 below)

2. If the infant is slowly dying; continued therapy only delays death

3. If the infant is and will probably remain unable to sustain itself

4. If continued therapy prolongs present pain

General "Human" Status

1. If the quality of life of the infant is and will be intolerable as judged by most reasonable persons: (the infant's life will predictably involve greater suffering than happiness and it will most probably be without self-awareness or socializing capacities)

2. If the infant will be totally handicapped and dependent

3. If the infant will be markedly impaired with small chance for normal existence

4. If the infant is defective and *unwanted* by its parents and unneeded by society

Question 2 cont'd

Medical Indications

1. If the infant has suffered irreparable damage to crucial organs, especially the brain

2. If the infant has meningomyelocele with no cord or bladder function

3. If the infant has hypoplastic (dysplastic) kidneys

4. If the infant is unable to be weaned from respirator

5. If the infant has a genetic defect linked to severe mental retardation requiring institutionalization

6. If the infant has hypoplastic lungs

7. If the infant has cardiac abnormalities for which no corrective or palliative treatment is possible

8. If the infant suffers from short gut syndrome

9. If the infant is anencephalic

LIMITING CONDITIONS: FAMILY SITUATION

(Note: All conditions listed here presuppose that the infant is severely defective)

1. If the survival of the infant would threaten the quality of life of the parents and the family as a whole

2. If the survival of the infant would impose excessive financial costs on the family

3. If the parents desire more speedy death for the dying infant

4. If the parents do not want to rear a severely handicapped child

5. If the parents are judged unable to nurture a severely handicapped infant

Question 2 cont'd

LIMITING CONDITIONS: MISCELLANEOUS

(Note: All conditions listed here presuppose that the infant is severely defective)

1. If the parents participate in the decision

2. If court arbitration is employed to resolve conflict between the physician and the family regarding the decision

3. If strong and continued support is available to parents who decide to have life support withdrawn

4. If there is an open and consistent nursery policy regarding such decisions

5. If the obligation to give care and comfort is understood to continue until death occurs

6. If the death of the infant would serve to overcome the demoralizing effect on the nursery staff of prolonged treatment of a hopeless case

QUESTION #3: WOULD IT EVER BE RIGHT TO INTERVENE DI-
RECTLY TO KILL A SELF-SUSTAINING INFANT?

ANSWERS: Yes 17[a]; No 2[b]; uncertain 1[c] *(further
comments listed below under Limiting
Conditions)*

LIMITING CONDITIONS: CHILD'S SITUATION

General Physical Status

1. If the infant is irretrievably dying a lingering
death

2. If the infant is dying painfully, or is in extreme pain or its life would be pain ridden

3. If the infant has gross physical anomalies

General "Human" Status

1. If the quality of life of the infant is and will
be intolerable as judged by most reasonable persons. The infant's life will predictably involve

---

[a] Many, especially the physicians, who responded "yes"
indicated that they would not intervene but would not
condemn another for doing so. Others indicated their
"yes" was intellectual, but they were emotionally un-
comfortable with the action.

[b] Two reasons cited: (a) *subjectively* impossible for re-
spondent; (b) only passive euthanasia is permissible.

[c] Uncertain because, although the act intends mercy, society seems wisely unwilling to approve of this kind of
power in the hands of physicians.

Question 3 cont'd

greater suffering than happiness and it will most probably be without self-awareness and socializing capacities

2. If the infant will be totally (or markedly) handicapped and dependent

3. If the infant is defective and unwanted by parents and unneeded by society

Medical Indications

1. If the infant is anencephalic

2. If the infant is hydrocephalic with little or no cortex

3. If the infant has massive brain damage

4. If the infant has a flat E.E.G.

5. If the infant has severe central nervous system disorders

6. If the infant has uncorrectable cardiac abnormalities, e.g., hypoplastic left heart syndrome

7. If the infant has Down's syndrome

8. If the infant has chromosomal disorders

9. If the infant has short gut syndrome

LIMITING CONDITIONS: FAMILY SITUATION

(Note: All conditions listed here presuppose that the infant is severely defective)

1. If the quality of parental life is threatened by continued survival of the infant

2. If the quality of familial life is threatened by the continued survival of the infant

3. If the parents desire the death of the infant

Question 3 cont'd

LIMITING CONDITIONS: MISCELLANEOUS

(Note: All conditions listed here presuppose that that the infant is severely defective)

1. If parents consent to the action

2. If the obligation to provide care and comfort is understood to continue to the moment of death

3. If the decision is understood to be the responsibility of the physician, advised by a neutral party, and the decision is made known to the parents

4. If *in loco parentis* the decision is made by the physician and a court appointed guardian

5. If, where feasible, there is prior review of the decision by a committee

6. If, where feasible, the responsible physician consults with an experienced colleague

7. If consideration is given to overcoming the demoralizing effect on the nursery staff of prolonged or cruel dying

8. If the means is chosen primarily because it offers the least painful death to the infant and secondarily because it offers least suffering to those around the dying infant

9. If the parents administered the syringe of KC1 prepared by the judge, and all the lawyers, priests, economists, psychologists, and journalists within a 50 mile radius as witnesses and no physicians, nurses or medical or nursing students were allowed to be present. (See also note 12, pp. 174-175.)

QUESTION #4: WOULD IT EVER BE RIGHT TO DISPLACE POOR PROGNOSIS INFANT A IN ORDER TO PROVIDE INTENSIVE CARE TO BETTER PROGNOSIS INFANT B?

ANSWERS: Yes 18; No 2[a] *(further comments listed below under Limiting Conditions)*

LIMITING CONDITIONS: CHILD'S SITUATION

General Physical Status

1. If there is a gross difference in prognosis between two infants

2. If infant A is *dying*, and infant B is truly viable (intact or nearly so)

3. If infant B would die without intensive care but otherwise has a good chance for intact survival

4. If infant A is in pain, has been treated for a reasonable period of time, and has certain prognosis for grossly abnormal life if he survives

General "Human" Status

1. If infant A would certainly have a poor quality, grossly abnormal life

2. If infant A has at best a 5% chance for meaningful existence

[a]Two reasons cited: (a) not a matter of morality but of practicality; no right/wrong; (b) policy favoring such action is too easily abused.

Question 4 cont'd

Medical Indications

1. If infant A is less than 1000 gm, has severe respiratory distress syndrome and has had a central nervous system bleed; and infant B is 1800 gm and has severe respiratory distress

2. If infant A is hopelessly toxoplasmic and infant B has neonatal tetanus

3. If infant A is older, exposed to prior stress, less mature and diagnosed as having presumed brain damage; and infant B is younger, more mature, and has no presumed brain damage

LIMITING CONDITIONS: FAMILY SITUATION

(Note: All conditions listed here presuppose that the infant is severely defective)

1. If infant A's survival would constitute a negative impact on its family's social and economic condition

LIMITING CONDITIONS: MISCELLANEOUS

(Note: All conditions listed here presuppose that the infant is severely defective)

1. If parental consent is obtained where possible

2. If certain POLICY MATTERS are operative:
a) some form of *prior review mechanism* is required (e.g., peer, arbitration panel, neutral party, court order)

b) there is *demonstrable certitude* that displacement is *necessary* to provide care for infant B and that there is a *vast difference in prognosis* for the two infants

c) the policy for allocating resources is clear, open and cautiously applied

d) there is a clear impartially applied formula for calculating who stands to gain the most from the therapy

Question 4 cont'd

3. If the situation is an *emergency*, the physician must decide and act on the basis of putting his efforts where they are likely to produce the greatest benefit to the greatest number

ADDITIONAL COMMENTS

1. This situation is not a *moral* problem but a tragic, necessary situation to be approached practically (like the life boat situation with too many wanting to get in). The *moral* problem would appear on the larger social scale if an affluent society permitted such needless, tragic scarcity to be chronic.

2. Displacement is *permissible* in this situation, but would not be so for adults who must be given security that they will not be bumped from life support machines to accommodate "better prognosis" latecomers.

INSTITUTE OF GOVERNMENTAL STUDIES

RECENT PUBLICATIONS

Monographs and Bibliographies

1976

Pers, Jessica S.
*Government as Parent: Administering Foster Care
in California.* 124pp $5.50

Wengert, Norman
*The Political Allocation of Benefits and Burdens:
Economic Externalities and Due Process in Environ-
mental Protection.* 43pp   2.50

1975

Pressman, Hope Hughes
*A New Resource for Welfare Reform: The Poor
Themselves.* 122pp   4.50

Scott, Stanley
Governing California's Coast. 454pp   9.75

1974

Lee, Eugene C. and Bruce E. Keith
*California Votes, 1960-1972: A Review and Anal-
ysis of Registration and Voting.* 172pp   7.50

1974 Supplement to California Votes, 1960-1972. 4pp   1.50

Gwyn, William B.
*Barriers to Establishing Urban Ombudsmen: The
Case of Newark.* 93pp   4.50

Tompkins, Dorothy C.
*Furlough From Prison. Public Policy Bibli-
ographies: 5.* 61pp   5.00

*Selection of the Vice President. Public Policy
Bibliographies: 6.* 26pp   3.75

Wyner, Alan J.
  The Nebraska Ombudsman: Innovation in State   6.75
  Government. 160pp

Working Papers

DeLeon, Richard and Richard LeGates
  Redistribution Effects of Special Revenue Sharing   2.50
  For Community Development. 59pp (June 1976)
  Working Paper #17

Jones, Victor, David Magleby, and Stanley Scott
  State-Local Relations in California. 81pp   2.50
  (October 1975) Working Paper #16

Radosevich, Ted C.
  Electoral Analysis of the Clean Water Bond Law of   2.50
  1974: Patterns of Support in a Continuing Environ-
  mental Issue. 75pp (August 1975) Working Paper #15

Public Affairs Report (selected issues)

Greenfield, Margaret and Alfred W. Childs, M.D.
  "Prepaid Health Plans: California's Experiment in
  Changing the Medical Care System" (April 1976)

Higgins, Tom
  "Juvenile Delinquency: Seeking Effective Prevention"
  (December 1975)

Starkweather, David B.
  "Hospitals: From Physician Dominance to Public Control"
  (October 1975)

Sherman, Patricia A.
  "Corrections: A Critical Analysis of the Prison System
  in California" (April 1975)

———

Send orders to the Institute of Governmental Studies, 109 Moses
Hall, University of California, Berkeley, CA 94720. Please
prepay orders for monographs, bibliographies and working papers.
California residents add 6% sales tax; residents of Alameda,
Contra Costa and San Francisco counties add 6 1/2% sales tax.

Single copies of the *Public Affairs Report* are free on request.